THE NATIONAL ADDICTION

Lies and Deception Disguised
As Mental Health

**How big drug companies,
politicians, and psychiatrists
create addiction and ignore real
treatments for mental health
problems**

Daniel J. Thompson, Ph.D.

ISBN 0615661297

ISBN-13   978-0615661292

Publisher: Laughing Mountain Publishing
            8600 Wurzbach Road, Suite 1103
            San Antonio, Texas 78240

To my wife, best friend, and editor,
Elizabeth, who celebrates life like a kitten
with a ball of twine. May you play
till the end of time.

CONTENTS

Preface

PART I   THE PROBLEM: A Society Headed for
                    Destruction from the Inside Out

PART II   THE PERFECT SOLUTION: The Only Way Out

Preface

Mental illness, particularly addiction, is not well understood by most of the people in the U.S. Many do not realize that addiction is by far the most prevalent and insidious aspect of mental illness in our society. Hopefully this book will provide a broad explanation of the addiction process and how it relates to mental health in general. I will explain how politicians, big drug companies, and medicine, through the actions of psychiatrists, disguise and distort mental illness into physical disease, and create addictions in the process of doing so. I want to provide some explanation of the common factors among addictions and other kinds of mental illness, as well as some explanation of the differences. At present the balance of our nation's mental health is severely threatened and growing worse. I feel moved to try to help inform others about this problem, and what can be done to change the growing chaos and destruction in our health system.

My major goal is to provide readers with information which can bring hope about recovery from addiction, as well as recovery from certain aspects of other mental illness. New research findings from science offer one of the most powerful tools for treatment ever to be discovered. There is exciting new hope for comprehensive treatment of the addictions as never before. My wish is that this book will motivate readers to continue to pursue legitimate mental health information and education for the sake of their own health, and also for others. If our society's present trend toward graft, deceit, and corruption in government and the health system is not reversed, our future looks grim. But, if enough of us learn to practice robust mental health, it can only result in peace and happiness. If we do this, our society and our nation will not only survive, it will thrive.

Peace,

Daniel

PART ONE

The Problem: A Society Headed for Destruction from the Inside Out

"For the great majority of mankind are satisfied by appearances, as though they were realities, and are often more influenced by the things that *seem* than by the things that are."

Niccolo' Machiavelli 1469-1527

1 THE NATIONAL ADDICTION

AN OVERVIEW

The United States is one of the most addicted societies on earth. Our society as a whole actually functions as a meta-addict. The roots of addiction are embedded deep in the American culture, although most people are oblivious to its growing presence. The society, and consequently our people, are addicted to any number of things and activities which are pathological in nature; but we don't seem to realize how extraordinarily dangerous this problem is. The underlying difficulty is that we do not seem to realize or understand what addiction actually is. When most people think of addiction, they usually think of other people they know who have been identified as alcoholics, or illegal drug addicts, or prescription drug addicts. Or perhaps they are reminded of the TV programs about celebrity recovery. However, most people will not think about themselves and their families and friends as addicts. But many of them already are; and many others of them will become pathological addicts if they continue along the same path that the society currently prescribes and encourages for them. There are many forms of addictive behaviors, which can be every bit as destructive as alcohol and drug addictions. These behavioral addictions are actually different facets of the same disease syndrome, the same as substance addictions, but we often minimize their danger or simply deny their severity. The most dangerous aspects of addiction are implicit in the multitude of ways our society twists, distorts, and corrupts our view of reality. All of our citizens have grown up in a culture which is so ingrained with addictive qualities that we now dismiss them as obvious, or simply shrug our shoulders, not recognizing the growing cancer in us. It will eventually cause the disintegration of our society, unless we deal with it. Addiction is not a moral issue *per se,* but is a disease process, which is like a parasite living internally, hidden inside our culture because it has become an everyday part of American life. The appetite of this growing parasite is voracious, and it has been growing for a very long time. In recent years it has become a pernicious monster, which eats at the very foundations of our nation and our most sacred principles. The fact that we do not recognize it or fear it is what makes us extremely vulnerable to its insidious destruction from the inside out. If we do not wake up and stop feeding this monster, it will devour us.

George, a financial manager for a large corporation, had been experiencing a somewhat bumpy period in his life. A crisis at work, though not really a critical one, demanded more work hours for its resolution than George was used to, and it demanded a lot of thought and study on his part. His wife Mary was not used to George's increased workload, although they both knew it was temporary. However, Mary's best friend had very recently moved out of town, and Mary was temporarily more dependent on George for attention than usual. These stressors, although both partners knew they were temporary and transient, had begun to interrupt George's sleep a little. In addition, he had not been getting his regular exercise, telling himself he could not afford the time to workout. Eating had become more irregular than usual, and he sometimes ate junk food, which he normally would avoid. A co-worker at the office, who had no knowledge of George's temporary stressors, mentioned to George that he seemed more anxious than usual. All this got George to thinking that maybe he should try to do something about his 'anxiety'. He had seen the commercials on TV, which talked about the feelings associated with anxiety and depression, and they recommended that certain medications may help with these symptoms. George considered his options. He could make an appointment with a psychiatrist and ask about medication.   Or, his internist already knew George so well that he would probably be willing to prescribe something without George having to go to a new doctor. George discounted the idea of counseling or psychotherapy with a psychologist (not a psychiatrist) immediately, because he didn't think there was any deep-seated problem that needed attention. Besides, therapy takes time, and he was sick and tired of being stressed and tired; he didn't want to wait. Also, he felt like he had no additional energy left over to make changes in his life while in the middle of this stressful period. So, George called his internist on the phone, who told George that he might be willing to prescribe something for him. But, the internist said that he would rather refer George to a psychiatrist for the 'right' medication, and that he could get him in to see the psychiatrist in a few days. Sure enough, George saw the psychiatrist, who after a long clinical interview, immediately prescribed an anti-anxiety medication for him. The medication did work to take the edge off the stress and to make George feel more 'mellow', in spite of the stresses in his life, which continued for several more weeks before returning to normal. George continued to take his medication even after the conditions at work and with Mary had returned to normal, because he liked the 'mellow' feeling. He told himself that, after all, he had to get his balance back gradually and gracefully. He also had noticed that the anti-anxiety medication was handy for using during the more irritating or boring times at work and home, such as the long rambling business meetings at work. They were mostly matters of tradition and not very interesting. He liked the ability to 'mellow-out' without others knowing what he was doing.

When George returned to the psychiatrist after two months for his medicine check, he was afraid that the doctor would not refill his prescription, since the period of stress in George's life was now essentially over. But, George had become accustomed to using the medication on an as-needs basis; and he really liked the feeling it gave him. It seemed to be a great remedy for a number of things, like anxiety, boredom, virtually any kind of stress, irritability, and general dissatisfaction. So, when faced with the psychiatrist's questions about how George was doing, George reported that he still needed the medication to deal with some stresses at work and at home. Yes, things were better, but not completely resolved yet. Consequently, the psychiatrist refilled George's prescription, and an addiction was born.

George's story is a typical example of how our society, and its commonplace actions, attitudes, and beliefs, misrepresent what mental health actually is, in order to sell us things. George's first inclination, as a result of the advertisements he had seen on TV, was to seek a pill, not real help to deal with stress from a counselor or psychotherapist. These advertisements, and the kind of medical bias they promote, substitute the idea that mental problems (even minor stresses) are medical problems instead of psychological problems. It disguises and reduces mental health issues into physical brain problems; and it suggests that the problems may be remedied with only a drug.

The television ads mentioned in George's story offer a prime example of how pharmaceutical companies encourage the distortion of mental health (and also other health issues) in order to sell more pills, and encourage drug addiction in the process. These commercials ask a few questions about a person's mood or behavior, and then *suggest* (*sell* is more accurate) that the person could have an actual mental disorder, and that their company's drug could be the appropriate treatment for this disorder (if it actually exists at all). The symptoms mentioned in the ad are almost always common, everyday emotions and behaviors experienced by almost everyone on the planet, at least occasionally (more on this in later chapters). The actual difficulty, like George's, is most often simply that life is sometimes uncomfortable. But that discomfort is usually transient; it most often passes when we take the necessary steps to change the situation. This is not to say that there are no legitimate mental illnesses, but mental health and mental illness exist on a continuum, they are not *things*; they refer to *processes*. Virtually all persons have been mentally ill, at least to some degree, at some point in their lives. However, most of us have not been *severely* mentally ill, and most people have *not* needed medication to heal. In most instances, exclusive reliance on medications keeps people from actually dealing with the real issues and instead keeps them focused on the symptoms. Psychoactive medications can only treat symptoms, not diseases or illnesses. They do not cure. *The essence of all addictions* is the distortion of reality to avoid dealing with the real issues. Psychologically, avoidance of the real issues of life is the sole purpose for the compulsive abuse of substances, actions, relationships, sex and many others things. The obvious consequence of addiction is that it does not solve the real difficulty.

Many (perhaps most) of our population seem to discount the importance of this problem, saying something like, "oh, this same thing has been around ever since the founding of our nation. Our free market system necessitates that buyers be aware that not everything they see on television ads will be right for them." This argument is legitimate, up to a point. But the central problem is the dishonesty about what mental health and mental illness actually are, and the cancerous general dishonesty growing in our culture.[1] There is a basic distortion of reality involved. It is perpetuated by the free market system, but is not a *necessary* component of the system. The ads referred to in George's story could be presented very differently and much more honestly. The pernicious societal delusion is driven by the *growing dishonesty in big business, the medical establishment, and government*, and, unfortunately, the passivity of the general population.[2] Consider for example, the so called *spin* used by advertisers and politicians to twist the truth in a particular direction. It usually involves only partial truths and sometimes even disregards essential truths. In defense of their actions, many pharmaceutical companies, politicians, and other big businesses often provide *more spin.* They usually are quick to explain away their words and actions as simply part of the traditional *free market philosophy*, inherent in our business and political culture. The fact is that we hear these bogus explanations so often, and they are so common, that people have come to take them for granted. We discount the danger, and believe there is no real problem. *This is not a free market philosophy; it is a lie.* When essential information is withheld, or advertisers create pseudo-problems in order to sell remedies, or they do not inform the public when there are much better proven remedies for health problems than those they offer, *they lie*. When politicians promise to be good and faithful representatives for their constituents, but actually spend their time, efforts, and influence for personal gain and for the special interest groups who back their campaigns, *they lie*. Democracy itself is undermined by dishonesty. It is sad to realize that this is politics as usual in the U.S., but *this is extremely destructive* **corruption.** To minimize its destructive results or call it anything less than *blatant dishonesty* is to participate in it and enable it.

The lies, or radically distorted truths, are especially destructive when they come from some of the largest and most prestigious institutions and companies in the country, including our own government. There are, of course, many fine and honorable business institutions and government officials, who act responsibly to stand on truth and integrity, and go out of their way to inform people of *necessary* information for their health and wellbeing. They are, as they should be, the standard bearers for the honest, courageous, and forthright America which we want to claim as our heritage. But, the increase of dishonesty, and the disregard of ideals in business and government is very severe and getting worse.

Added to the abuses and addictions created by dishonest commercials pushing prescription drugs, and dishonest government supporting the deceptions, are the enormous quantities of alcohol and illegal drugs which are consumed in our society. Alcohol and drug abuse counselors report that their clients almost always say that they are abusing the addictive substances to 'medicate' their anxiety, pain, depression, stress, or obsessive thinking. The essence of addictive behaviors is the motivation to *change everyday reality*, because everyday reality is perceived as intolerable. The only reason to continue to use any drug until it becomes an addiction is that the person *prefers* the feelings the substance offers over everyday reality. For instance, George's burgeoning addiction to a *legal* drug follows all of the same psychological principles and processes as an *illegal* drug addiction. This resistance to everyday reality results, for the addict, in chronic anxiety, depression, stress, and/or obsessive thinking. Regardless of how the drug dependence gets started, the addiction is perpetuated by the rationalizations of the addict, telling him/her self that he or she *needs* to keep taking the drug in order to feel 'okay'. The person is driven to try to reduce the symptoms by whatever means. Addiction is *escapism*, but the attempt to escape makes things even worse. Eventually the addict may not remember accurately what she/he was trying to escape from in the first place. What was, in the beginning, escape from *specific* things, people, responsibilities, or issues, has eventually turned into escape from *everything*, including everyday life.

We Americans live in what is probably the most addictive society in the world. Any system, no matter how large or complex, can act as an addict.[3] Our societal addiction arises from our materialism; we tend to *thingify* the world (conceptualize reality as things). Addiction is created by the delusion that reality can be reduced to things and superficial activities. It is the *avoidance* of real life-meaning by focusing on things, images, and the superficial aspects of life. Addiction tries to avoid dealing with life on life's terms, and it always fails. It leaves the addict craving real life-meaning, but frustrated in his or her attempts to get it, because she or he has been taught by the society (TV, magazines, etc.) that things alone should provide it. So the person chases more things, drugs, alcohol, sex, or shallow relationships, anything that provides a diversion. That is addiction. The compulsive repetition of the same behaviors over and over, hoping for different results, is the symptom; the actual disorder is the *distorted view of reality*.

The common denominator between addiction, the distorted view of mental health, and the avoidance of reality is that they all perpetuate the practice of irresponsibility and deceit. This eats at the very core of our national integrity. Case in point is the fact that the U.S. seems to be losing the admiration and respect of the rest of the world like an avalanche slipping into the sea. A major part of this is due to dishonesty. Consider the justification given for invading Iraq based on bogus 'weapons of mass destruction', said to be a hidden threat to the world, supposedly located somewhere in Iraq. How can this terrible dishonesty be justly rationalized away as poor judgment or mismanagement of information on the part of the government administration? The American government lied to the whole world.[4] After that, not to mention the many other atrocities committed by our government on foreign soil, it would be ludicrous to expect that other nations will respect us for our integrity. Big business and government, with the majority of our population following like lemmings, somehow are trying to tell themselves and the rest of the world that it is possible to be sane and dishonest at the same time. This is an absolute contradiction. Sanity cannot be expected to prevail in an unpredictable environment of dishonesty.

Drugs will not fix dishonesty, and they are a very dangerous substitute. Mental problems cannot be legitimately reduced to a simple set of labels or diagnoses, which describe medical diseases; nor can their treatment be reduced legitimately to the administration of drugs. Mental illnesses, even in those cases with heavy genetic loading and/or demonstrable brain involvement are not succinct, clearly defined diseases, the same from person to person. Rather, they are complex life processes, for which the same diagnosis (syndrome) often varies greatly from person to person. Labels such as *depression, anxiety, obsessive-compulsive thoughts and behavior, mood swings, neurotic avoidance,* and others are, first of all, *common characteristics of normal human emotions and behaviors*, which are usually resolved with the appropriate action and the passage of some reasonable time period. However, the *Diagnostic and Statistical Manual* [5] produced by the American Psychiatric Association is the medically accepted Bible for the diagnosis of mental and psychiatric disorders in the U.S. This book is produced almost exclusively by physicians, due to the huge political power of the American Medical Association; and it lists every one of the common human characteristics listed above, including many others, as *mental disorders*, not just extreme cases of common human characteristics. Even some behaviors, like shyness for example, are given such labels as *social phobia*, and are claimed to be psychiatric problems, which can be treated with drugs (more on this in later chapters). Such materialistic thinking attempts to reduce the world to black and white decisions; as if a person either has the symptoms or he/she doesn't have them. It is necessary to *thingify* emotions and behaviors in order to sell drugs to treat them. Reality is reduced to content instead of process. The greed of our frenetic society, with its bent for reducing the world to things, its rush to oversimplify reality, and its huge motivation to commercialize almost everything, advertises pills for symptoms typical of nothing more than a bad day. This is not to say that severe problems, which actually need the benefit of medication, do not exist. We should be very thankful to have such medications, and the medical personnel to administer them. But, it is the greed of some pharmaceutical companies, and even the medical system itself, which often distorts the treatment of mental problems into an extremely shortsighted and dangerous practice. It's like selling wart removal remedies or Band-Aids for mental and emotional difficulties. This same kind of thinking is also responsible for the government's lack of funding for legitimate mental health care and prevention programs. Add to this the government's 'war on drugs'. Consider the vast expense and the atrocious loss of lives due to this government fiasco, not to mention the huge number of lives ruined by incarceration for simple possession of drugs with no intent to distribute. We could be funding a 'war on addiction' (treatment of addicts) with the same money (very likely would need less money) and save virtually all of the lives lost as a result of our present drug policy. The societal delusion here is that the *drugs* being abused are seen as the problem. The real problem is the *addiction* of the people abusing the drugs, and that addiction is what needs to be treated.

There may be some temptation at this point to assume that it is mere ignorance and naiveté on our part. Perhaps the average person (including the government) simply doesn't understand addiction and mental health. While there may be a modicum of truth to that idea, this is the kind of thinking that is known, in mental health terms, as *denial*. The fact is, many people in our society don't want to face the responsibility necessary for dealing with the real truth. Philosopher/economist George Soros says, "what is wrong with America? People are not particularly concerned with the pursuit of truth. They have been conditioned by ever more sophisticated techniques of manipulation to the point where they do not mind being deceived; indeed, they seem positively to invite it".[6] And the sickest part of this scenario is that big business, often in collusion with government, *wants us to continue to deny our responsibility* for dealing directly with the issues. They apparently believe that the economy is dependent on it.[7] They apparently believe that we must continue to *consume more and more things*, whether they are necessary or not, regardless of whether the ads are truthful or not. This is the same kind of rationale which set up the recent national economic crisis based on the overextension of credit. Hopefully our people are beginning to learn that, when big banks and mortgage companies pander to needy people who cannot yet afford to buy homes, they lie. They suggest to them that, "yes we can qualify you for a loan, just sign here". Everyone involved participates in *clinical denial* at least, if not conscious criminal intent. Everyone involved participates in a lie, almost certain to lead to negative consequences. It is imperative that our people recognize that the same scenario is occurring in the field of mental health, with a huge potential for disastrous results. Our society has backed itself into a corner where it teaches addiction as a treatment for mental health problems, because the so-called 'treatment' is quick and simple; so what if it is overly expensive, short-sighted, and often ignores the real issues having to do with honesty and personal responsibility. All that the person needs to do is side-step the real issues and take another pill or a drink (because a pill *really is* necessary to damp the bad feelings which result from dishonesty, avoidance of responsibility, failure to admit guilt when appropriate, and the lack of courage to do what is right). That is addiction in action. Again, this is not to say that there aren't legitimate reasons for the use of medications for mental problems. But, the society as a whole is not just inching toward a collective case of neurotic blindness; it is running headlong toward the disintegration and abandonment of personal and cultural values on which our nation was founded.

Peace is the true remedy for mental health problems. When most people hear the word peace, they immediately assume the speaker is talking about international peace. But, *peace*, personal, interpersonal, societal, and international begins at the level of the *individual*. Individual personal peace implies contentment, at least for the moment; and those who practice it regularly associate it with happiness. Which comes first, happiness or peace? The typical answer is happiness, but the correct answer is peace. Peace is a choice, not a response. It is a state of being we can make happen, not the result of everything outside of ourselves being in order. But peace cannot be had without responsibility. We must, first of all, take *primary* responsibility for the management of our own personal health issues, physical, mental, and spiritual. This is not a suggestion for the imposition of some new sort of societal order; it is a *natural* fact that the only person I can change is my self. No other human knows the intricacies and complexities of an individual better than him/her self. We are each responsible for managing our own health in the same way we are responsible for getting food and cleaning ourselves. It is not just a privilege; it is a *necessity* to take on this responsibility. We cannot simply abdicate this responsibility by deferring it to others. Of course, we must use health consultants, including physicians, dentists, psychologists, and others, for both treatment and prevention; we definitely need the benefit of their expertise. But, we cannot expect, in a culture where *buyer beware* is the standard mantra, that others will automatically take adequate care of us just because they have medical or pharmacy degrees. Each of us must always hold and keep the *primary* responsibility for our own health, and always remember that health professionals are only our consultants and specialists, to serve at our bidding.

The duty of doctors and health care professionals of virtually every kind is *not* to tell us what to do. Doctors should, first of all, be teachers and explain to us what our treatment options are. The health professional should never presume that he or she, and what they have to offer, will automatically be the patient's treatment of choice. A healthy skepticism is recommended when choosing and using health care professionals. Any doctor who assumes the he or she and their recommendations are above question is too arrogant to be trusted. Patients should ask lots of questions about their doctor's credentials and experience, the proposed treatments, and anything else that the patient needs to know in order to make good health decisions. Any doctor who seems the least bit frustrated with questions from the patient should not be trusted. To the contrary, health care professionals should welcome and invite questions. There are many fine professionals who will do just that. The first responsibility of health care professionals is to help patients and clients learn what their options are, and how to compare them.

People, businesses, and institutions who distort the truth, including many advertisers, big businesses, politicians, and others do not want to be questioned about what they say and do. Commerce rules our world, and unfortunately, advertisers can lie and distort the truth to sell more products. We *should* question them in whatever way we can. And when we get answers that are off the point, too general to be useful, or diversions designed to lead us away from the question, we should find other products, politicians, or businesses who offer reasonable information. None of us are immune to the insidious distortions of the truth perpetuated by big business, the government, and the news media. In today's world, virtually every day's news is punctuated by huge scandals in government and business, all having to do with dishonesty. But the corruption of mental health is much more insidious and indirect. All of us, as a society, are responsible for perpetuating this collective suicide mission.

The only way out is to take charge of our selves individually, and to practice rigorous honesty with our selves and others. Most of the so-called 'mental health problems' in our nation would never arise if people were willing to be rigorously honest with their selves and others. Indeed, most psychotherapists and mental health counselors spend the majority of their time trying to get people to *want* to change. The issue is usually not that people are consciously dishonest, but that they believe their own lies, and are blinded by the illusions, hype, spin, and outright false statements that are often spread by even the medical industry itself. In terms of mental health, our society teaches people to believe they are helpless. It teaches that mental health is a commodity. To get it, you have to buy it; what does personal responsibility have to do with it? We have begun to believe the lies told by the advertisers. But, most mental health issues cannot be accurately characterized as diseases. *Self-deception* is the primary ingredient of most mental problems. Honest *self-awareness* is the key ingredient of mental health.

There is a true remedy available for this malignancy in our society. It does start with personal peace, but the groundwork for personal peace is rigorous honesty, and the willfulness and courage to do the most constructive thing possible for everyone's benefit, when faced with a choice of actions. There is a wonderful secret, seemingly a paradox, which the addicted person (and our society as a meta-addict) seems not to know. It is that the energetic pursuit of self awareness, honesty, and personal responsibility will not only remedy most of the problems; they will result in true happiness, personal peace, rich life meaning, and healthy loving relationships, the very things the addict has been craving. However, for a large percentage of our population, the addictive veil of avoidance and escapism keeps them from recognizing that this is actually possible. True addiction has set in, and the addiction is pervasive and insidious; it has become addiction to the world of *things* in general. Although the addict may have one or more primary addictions, such as drugs, alcohol, spending, sex, codependent relationships, etc., the addiction syndrome is played out in virtually every facet of the person's life. It has become an addiction precisely because the person believes only in things. In this addictive state, even the self and other people are thought of merely as things to manipulate to try to find some kind of satisfaction. Although many people pay lip service to spiritual or religious issues, or to loving relationships, for many their true beliefs and attitudes are locked into the flat cause-and-effect reasoning of the *thing* world. But any satisfaction based totally on things is always transient and temporary. The addictive system is inherently dishonest, because it is out of touch with reality. It diminishes reality to its lowest common denominator, material things.

True mental health is holistic balance at the mental, physical, and spiritual levels. True mental health encourages raising our level of conscious awareness to include as much of reality as possible. Addiction necessitates that we deny any aspects of reality (keep them as unconscious as possible), which might be uncomfortable or unpleasant or simply unwanted. The addict is in a jail created by him/her self personally. The addict remains captive because he/she simply doesn't believe that life would be tolerable without the things around them to provide a buffer against natural reality. True mental health, looking at life with eyes wide open, sets us free. Freedom can be had only with the practice of rigorous honesty, responsibility, and peace. True mental health will allow us and our nation not just to survive, but to *thrive.*

2

WHAT IS MENTAL HEALTH?

George continued to take his anti-anxiety medication, and was pleased that it worked so well to reduce his stress, boredom, irritability, and unrest of virtually every kind that entered into his life. He had been taking it on an as-needs basis for a number of months, and was very accustomed to the way it worked. All he had to do, if the effect wore off, is take another pill. However, he had noticed that it seemed to take more pills to keep him happy as time wore on. But he was relatively tranquil virtually all of the time. Life seemed easier. But, George was getting bored. His life seemed to have no verve, not enough excitement. It seemed like all he did was work at a job which was tolerable, but very routine; then he went home and watched TV or surfed the internet.   His energy felt lower than he wanted it to be. George had begun to back off of his exercise routine, which used to be a regular thing. He had no hobbies, and he seldom spent time with friends except at work. His relationship with Mary was okay, but also very routine. He wished something exciting would happen, but seemed helpless to initiate anything for himself. It was as if something would have to happen *to* him, from outside himself, in order for things to change. George had also begun to notice that the pills had become more and more of a need, not just a luxury anymore. When he tried to go without them, he became anxious, irritable, and unhappy.

Fortunately, after several more weeks had passed, George began to get consciousness enough to realize that he was, indeed, addicted. He had very little in his life that he considered meaningful, except the pills. He told himself that he had to get a real life. After a few more days he mustered the courage to call his psychiatrist and make an appointment. George did, in fact, go to the appointment, and told his psychiatrist that he wanted to stop using the pills, but that he didn't know how to do it. He just couldn't seem to accomplish it on his own. The doctor told George that he was fortunate that he had not tried to stop abruptly, all at once; because there is significant risk of seizures occurring when someone tries to do that. The psychiatrist suggested that George could try another drug, but George was wise enough to refuse. So, the psychiatrist put George on a tapering schedule, so that George would use smaller and smaller doses of his present medication over the course of about six weeks. Then he would be free. Also, the doctor was wise and experienced enough to recommend that George might want to get some psychotherapy or counseling, in case he had difficulty withdrawing from the medication. He gave George the name and number of a clinical psychologist. George followed the doctor's orders exactly and tapered off of the medication until he had no more left. It was difficult, because very little else had changed in George's life, except he was a little more 'edgy'. Nevertheless, he was in fact free of his dependence on the medication. But, George did not go to the psychologist, as the doctor had recommended, because he did not see the relevance. He just needed to stop the medication, and he did. But George's unrest and discontent did not go away.

The World Health Organization defines mental health as, "a state of well-being in which the individual realizes his or her own abilities, can cope with the normal stresses of life, can work productively and fruitfully, and is able to make a contribution to his or her community". [8] There are, of course, slightly different emphases for different cultures, but the definition above fits our own culture rather well. So, why is defining mental health so important? The answer is that, mental health is one of those things that is easy to take for granted when we are happy. It is similar to other kinds of health, in that we assume we have health when we do not see or feel signs of illness. In other words, the concept of mental health is dependent on the concept of mental illness for its definition, at least to some degree. However, there is much more to the concept of mental health than the lack of symptoms of mental illness; and this is the very point at which pharmaceutical companies, the government, and the medical industry itself sneak in to sell our citizens addiction in place of real mental health. Notice that the World Health Organization definition above does not talk about mental health as a thing, or a black/white, on/off phenomenon. Instead, it outlines *processes*, actions, cognitions, feelings, and behaviors. Mental health exists on a continuum ranging from a lot to a little, not like an on/off switch. Mental health is an ongoing process. Most people, at some point in their lives, have been mentally ill for a few hours or for a few days. However, the problem most often is transient and temporary. Often simply the passing of time resolves it. But, in our society mental health/illness is often assumed to follow the same principles we use for physical problems. It does not. This difference, in how mental health is viewed, is also the crux of the problem our society has with addictions. Addictions have a lot to do with on/off and black/white thinking, and *thingifying* the world. There is confusion about the meaning of addiction in the same way there is confusion about other mental health issues. Mental illness and addiction must not be treated like physical disease; the issues are much broader.

In regard to physical health, a physician, when asked to explain how to stay adequately healthy and to avoid hospitalizations once said, "don't go to your doctor any more than is really necessary".[9] This doctor, a competent, kind, and compassionate family physician, was pointing out that, traditionally, the only thing a person will get if he visits his/her physician is a recommendation for *treatment* or *testing*. The typical physician does not assume that people will visit him or her to learn about health, but only to get treatment for illness. This assumption, that we are well unless we have symptoms, is the basis for the kind of medicine practiced in the U.S. Western medical theory relies heavily on the principle of *homeostasis,* or balance in the body. It theorizes that the *livingness* of an organism is maintained by its natural automatic ability to bring itself back into balance when stressed. For instance, the human body automatically regulates its own internal temperature, maintaining it at a consistent level which varies only slightly even under extreme external conditions. Likewise, healing from a physical wound is the process of homeostasis, as the body moves back toward equilibrium. This theory of life leads us to assume that there is no reason to visit a physician unless we have some problem we can point out.

Maintaining good physical health does demand that people practice certain good health habits, but these traditionally have been aimed at the *avoidance* of contaminants and injurious situations. Only fairly recently has our society begun to emphasize, in earnest, the necessity for *proactive* preventive measures such as regular exercise, good nutrition, etc. Generally speaking, we have been taught to rely on the natural homeostasis of the body to keep us healthy physically. However, we cannot rely on natural homeostasis to keep us *mentally* healthy. Mental health, much more so than physical health, necessitates the conscious practice of good habits involving virtually every facet of our lives. Good mental health involves huge amounts of learning and acculturation. Rigorous honesty, accepting personal responsibility, willingness to share, a desire to relate to others equitably, belief in the value and meaningfulness of life, a wish to contribute to life, and a general willingness to live life on life's terms, are all necessary components of good mental health. Life balance is obviously a good measuring stick for mental health. However, unlike homeostasis, this necessary balance is not automatic and unconscious. It necessitates continual *conscious* awareness, willingness, and effort to maintain equilibrium. There are very many facets of our existence to keep in balance; for example, work and play, self and others, emotions and intellect, routine and creativity, and mind-body-spirit, just to mention a few. Mental health necessitates conscious, deliberate thinking, and planning, willfulness, action, and peacefulness. Staying free of addictions, as part of mental health, needs this same kind of conscious, proactive attention to good health habits and balance. We must not assume that natural homeostasis will lead us back to an addiction-free state. In our hyper-materialistic, acquisition-obsessed, competitive society, the most likely default state may be addiction.

Our mental health has everything to do with happiness. Real happiness may be the best yardstick of all for measuring mental health, because a person with *real* happiness feels good about self and others; she or he does not harbor guilt or resentment; she or he loves life; and is constructive and playful. These qualities cannot be gotten with a pill. They are the result of good intentions, decent choices, and requisite actions. It is true, of course, that physical health, genetics, brain chemistry, and other factors may play a significant role in the mental health of some people. However, for almost everyone, mental health is primarily mediated by the *mind*, not just the brain. The mind cannot be simply reduced to brain function, because the mind is a composite of choices, habits, beliefs, attitudes, fears, desires, emotions, memories, goals, and self-aware meaningfulness, issues, things, generalities, and abstractions which are far too complex to be mediated by the physical brain alone (more about mind vs. brain in later chapters).

George was now free of the anxiety medication, but virtually nothing else in his life had changed. He began to wonder what had really motivated him to start the medication in the first place. True, he had been responding to stress, but the stress itself had actually been only mild to moderate, and he had known that it would pass within a few weeks. It seemed odd because he now realized that he was and had been *bored* most of the time. It was as if he was stressed by boredom and routine. George decided that he must be missing something. He was not really happy, but he couldn't really say that he had any significant mental health problems. He just was not happy enough. Perhaps he should have taken the psychiatrists advice and gone to see a psychotherapist. He made an appointment with a clinical psychologist.

George talked to the psychotherapist, and they established a working relationship. The basic contract that the therapist proposed was that, if George would take on the responsibility of defining and describing himself to the therapist as thoroughly as possible, the therapist would take on the responsibility of helping George try on some different 'hats', which might fit. These 'hats' might be possible explanations for George's emotions and behaviors, or they might be suggestions about how George could possibly do things differently. George liked this contract. It reassured him that he was in charge of making any decisions for his life, and that the psychologist was simply a diligent consultant, nothing more/nothing less, a specialist in the exploration of the psyche. George started out seeing the therapist once each week for an hour, and his interest and curiosity about himself grew as they proceeded. Within a few sessions, the therapist had explained to George that the everyday standards for mental health espoused by our society are very superficial and short-sighted in many ways. George began to realize that, in spite of the fact that he had achieved virtually everything we associate with success and happiness in our society (although he was not wealthy, he made a decent income and was financially secure, he had a pleasant marriage to someone he loved, he owned the "right" things, etc.), he was not really satisfied with his life. He felt he had no real meaning. So, George began to realize that real mental health is something bigger than not having huge problems to deal with. It does have to do with the idea of happiness, motivation, zest for life, fun, and an idea of life's meaning to fit his unique self. He also began to realize, with the therapist's help, that there could be no real happiness without rigorous honesty. He had to get his slate clean and keep it clean. That way, he never had to hide from himself or anyone else. Not with false pride, but with true humility, he could relate to the rest of the world as equals. His internal playing field would always be level, and he could trust himself to be straight with everyone and to accept only the same in return. The fact that real mental health is so dependent on moral and ethical considerations is the main difference. There is a tendency for each of us, like small children, to want to avoid responsibility or to take the easy way out. But, as most grownups are aware, there is a substantial payoff for acting responsibly as adults, such as being known as a safe and trustworthy person, being able to keep a job, successfully relating to loved ones, and building the kind of life we aspire to in the real world. It is definitely a matter of balancing short-term and long-term goals. The issue of ethics and morals is such a common basic concern that we often don't see the need to consider it when we think of health. In addition, we also know that being honest, trustworthy, and responsible are not black/ white concepts. As a matter of fact, it is impossible for any person to be *perfectly* honest, trustworthy, etc. Sometimes people make destructive choices because they do not have enough information to make constructive ones. No person can consistently and accurately predict the future. This is what we mean by the *development of good judgment*. We have all had to *learn* to be honest and responsible as we grew into maturity. And many of us were told, growing up, that it is *necessary* to tell 'white lies', in order to be polite and not hurt other people's feelings. These considerations are so fundamental to our societal order that adults often simply take them for granted, forgetting that truth is the basic necessity for discerning reality. Even mental health counselors often pay too little attention to honesty, assuming that clients surly will realize the necessity of being truthful with their therapists and the rest of the world. However, addiction specialists deal with the denial and dishonesty of their clients routinely, and they do expect the question of honesty to be a major issue in therapy. Ideally, all therapists, clinicians, counselors, and indeed all of our population should realize and be vigilant about rigorous honesty. Truth is the most fundamental necessity for mental health and for the avoidance/treatment of addictions. It is an appalling fact of American life today that our government, big business, big pharmaceutical companies, and the medical health industry are teaching our population to practice dishonesty by what they do and say. It is sad, but nevertheless true, that we as individuals must choose to be honest for ourselves, even though our most powerful leaders often do not offer a model of honesty for us to follow. Many of our most powerful would-be leaders do not teach health, they teach illness and addiction. We must, for the sake of survival, be extremely skeptical of their words and actions. If we do not, we will automatically be infected by them, like a virus infects a computer. We should realize that dishonesty is more and more pervasive in our culture as time goes on. More things (or pills) will not remedy the avoidance of reality created by dishonesty. Nor will filling up our lives with more frenetic activity satisfy our longing for peace and serenity. We must stop and listen to what reality has to tell us. We must *choose* peace; it has to be purchased with honest living, and being in the present with life on life's terms.

Many of us have grown up in an atmosphere of chaos and crisis and never have experienced real peace. This actually makes some people afraid of peace, because they are afraid of the unknown. Some people are afraid to stop and be still. Often, they associate peace with nothingness. It can sometimes take courage to still the mind and actually *listen* to the silence and to what it has to teach us. Robust mental health necessitates being totally willing to see ourselves and the world around us for who and what we really are, without having an internal dialogue running at the same time. The goal is to sense ourselves in our natural state of being without talking about it while we are trying to do it. Occasionally, in order to know ourselves, we must focus all of our attention on *being* without *doing.*

By now, it should be obvious that mental health is a balanced composite of all of the feelings, behaviors, attitudes, and beliefs which make us into adaptive human beings. It is an ongoing process, which must endure ups and downs and stresses and joys and disappointments and all that life brings our way. We cannot expect to be mentally healthy and in balance simply by going along with the rest of society. We have to make individual and personal choices that assure our own health, irrespective of the society at large.

The mental health of our younger generations is more at risk in some ways. They have been born into the huge influence of dishonesty and misinformation to be found on the internet and other electronic media sources. Almost every day we read or hear about some internet stalking, victimization, or other criminal activity involving the naiveté and gullibility of youngsters. In addition, a virtual alternative culture is proliferated by some internet games, fantasy websites and bulletin boards, pernicious gossip, paranoid conspiracy theories, and immoral, unethical, and sometimes criminal manipulations on the internet. The internet adds to dishonesty simply because it provides *more* exposures to all kinds of information all the time, a significant proportion of which are lies and distortions of the truth. The internet also engenders its own special brand of delusion, which places our youth and some adults at increased risk. This kind of delusion is due to the fantasy-like reality which some electronic and internet games encourage, and the detached, machine-like, relationship-at-a-distance interactions between people on the internet. Internet addiction itself has become one of the most dangerous kinds of addiction in our society, because it reduces reality simply to so many clicks on a mouse or keyboard. On the internet, there are no *real* people to be found; only words and images projected onto a screen. It is easy to learn to depersonalize others (turn them into things), when one learns to relate to them only from an electronic distance.

Mental illness, of course, assumes that some of the factors which we associate with mental health, such as emotional balance, reasonable judgment, capacity for constructive relationships, and others, are not currently functioning well. However, as mentioned above, mental health is much more than the relative absence of mental illness. A person who practices and usually maintains good mental health may find him or her self in a temporary (or longer) out-of-balance situation, which could be diagnosed as a mental problem. Some psychologists and other mental health professionals prefer just to call mental health problems, *problems of living.* This signification, *problems of living*, points to the fact that life itself, even at best, presents obstacles and stresses to deal with. The goal of mental health is to learn to negotiate these bumps in the road of life with as much peace, balance, and as adaptively as possible. The goal of life should not be to try to avoid problems which are unavoidable, but to deal with problems effectively without letting them knock us out of balance.

Mental problems, first of all, regardless of whether they are large or small, temporary or longer term, result from *stressors.* The primary stressors can be physical, mental, or spiritual, or can involve all three facets at to some degree. Physical stressors, of course, involve many kinds of physical disease, disability, loss of capacity, chronic physical syndromes, and also brain diseases or dysfunctions. Mental stressors which do not involve the brain directly are those problems of living which include dealing with the environment outside our selves, loss, grief, problem solving, judgment, short-term coping skills, and most often, interpersonal relationships, among others. Spiritual stressors involve life meaning, life goals, and other big-picture aspects of life, including religious aspects. By far, the majority of problems of life, which get labeled as mental problems, fall in the category of *mental* issues as opposed to physical issues. The spiritual aspect is involved implicitly, simply because it is inherent in everything.

The huge mistake made so often by medical psychiatry, although it appears clear and simple to most people when they understand how it works, is that psychiatry treats virtually *every* kind of problem of living as a physical problem. There are, to be sure, those *physical* brain problems which sometime result in inappropriate, difficult, psychotic, or possibly destructive feelings and actions. They desperately need the medications provided by psychiatrists. These brain-involved, chronic, and sometimes severe mental problems can be very difficult to deal with. They need the finest medical attention psychiatry has to offer, but they also almost always need psychological treatment from a psychotherapist. However, psychiatry itself often distorts reality and *adds to everyday problems*, teaching the patient an incorrect view of reality. This happens when the problems (by far most problems) fall in the *mental* and *spiritual* categories. Psychiatry doesn't seem to be able to overcome its flawed and antiquated bias which assumes that everything in the world is physical or material. This flawed philosophy of science persists, in spite of the fact that there has never been any scientific evidence explaining how an imbalance of chemicals in the brain actually causes psychological problems. [10] In addition, for comprehensive treatment of mental problems to occur, psychotherapy or counseling should be recommended in *most* cases, even in those cases where medication is necessary, or where the problems are primarily physical. Psychotropic medications usually do not actually cure problems, they only temporarily alter the symptoms; and most often there are side effects. [11] However, psychotherapy focuses on teaching clients new coping skills, how to handle emotions constructively, and relationship skills, knowledge and behaviors which do, indeed, help people to live adaptively, and without any side effects. A good rule of thumb is that almost all problems of living are best treated with some amount of psychotherapy or counseling; and some of these problems (fewer) will benefit additionally from medication. However, a safety-first rule should always be considered; if a person is actively hallucinating or acting psychotic, self-injurious or homicidal, they should always be referred to a medical emergency facility immediately. Sometimes help from law enforcement officers may be necessary. The reason for this should be obvious; medical facilities and physicians are the primary administrators of medications and of in-patient treatment care facilities which offer the safety of 24-hour care. In emergency cases, these facilities and personnel are necessary to keep people from harming themselves and others. Psychotropic medications are almost always needed in these instances.

3
WHAT IS ADDICTION?

Addiction is not well understood by most of the people in our society. Among addiction specialists and researchers the word *addiction* is often avoided because it has such a wide range of meanings, including physiological dependence, psychological dependence, chronic abuse, and various arguments concerning whether the word should only apply to substances as opposed to behaviors, such as sex addiction, codependence, food addiction, etc. However, in recent years it has been discovered that many different activities, including all of the above, and other such behaviors as compulsive video gaming, compulsive texting, compulsive gambling, compulsive exercising, and others all have a common brain component which links them as addictions. All of these repetitive compulsive behaviors hijack the brain's pleasure pathways, the same ones activated with hard drugs, and cause withdrawal symptoms when the behaviors are stopped arbitrarily.[12] Just like drugs, these compulsive behaviors result in a *high,* which includes euphoria, anxiety reduction, and sometimes even dissociation from the surrounding environment. In truth, all of the above are 'hard' addictions. Abrupt withdrawal from the excessive behavior often results in increased anxiety, irritation, confusion, and severe discomfort for the addict, essentially the same as withdrawal from drugs, but without the same degree of physiological involvement. However, it appears to the average person to be merely a lack of character or moral fiber on the addict's part. The typical person who is not addicted believes the addict should simply choose to stop it (if I can stop when I want to, why can't you?).   But, the critics of substance abusers are sometimes addicted themselves to other substances or activities, including work, sex, sports, the internet, or even people, just to mention a few, not recognizing that these other behaviors can also become hard addictions. Nevertheless, the substance addict is generally thought of in critical terms, as weak and unable to control him/her self. After the addiction has been active for some length of time, the addict will inevitably have gotten the message from others, that they believe the addict uses too much or behaves inappropriately. The addict typically responds by trying to control the amount of the substance or activity used, but often fails. When the addict fails, he or she feels *shame,* and begins to worry that maybe his or her critics are right; perhaps he or she is too weak or somehow different than normal humans.[13] At first, the psyche of the addict is very resistant to accepting the idea that something may be inherently defective in his or her character. The addict's psychological defenses make him or her want to fight off the critics and avoid any new criticism. Often, in reaction, the addict him/herself will become a zealous critic of others' actions in an attempt (usually unconsciously) to keep her/himself off of the hot seat. Like the old game of 'hot potato', the addict wants to move the attention to someone else. Therefore, he or she becomes a proactive and preemptive critic of others' actions and words. We are all familiar with the stereotypic image (usually in the movies) of the cynical and bitter drunk who blames everyone else for everything. Needless to say, the addict denies to others that he/she might have a problem. The addict feels that she/he did not invite the runaway use of the alcohol, drug, food, activity or other substance; he or she just can't seem to stop it or moderate its use to a reasonable level. We sometimes overlook the fact that no person (other than someone intent on suicide) would decide consciously to become or remain an addict, because eventually the addiction results in rejection, pain and misery. But the addiction is like a parasite which will not let go of the host. Often times, even if the addict manages to stop abusing one substance, she or he may begin abusing another addictive substance or activity. Also, if a person manages to *force* him/her self to quit, but does not change anything else in his or her life, the 'dry' addict usually remains a bitter, resentful, or unhappy person. This occurs because the origins of the addiction, and the other life factors which help to perpetuate the addiction, have not been addressed. The person in that situation has managed arbitrarily to remove the symptom, but has not dealt with the disease. This is why a substitute addiction may be adopted to replace the original forbidden substance.

George had stopped going to see the psychologist. He had to admit that he understood all that the psychologist said, and it did sound logical. But he didn't believe wholeheartedly that the changes recommended could actually result in the happiness the therapist held out as the goal of treatment. It sounded a little too idealistic for George. He was not really sure that anyone actually ever attained that kind of peace and meaningfulness in life. George considered the actions and words of his friends and business associates, and the significant people he had known. While some of them *professed* to be happy, like the psychologist had said, those who were really successful by our society's standards (generally the wealthy and powerful), appeared untouched by real life. Virtually all of them seemed somewhat superficial and unburdened by the everyday problems and responsibilities most people have to live with. The rich and powerful hired other people to take care of those things. They appeared to be surrounded by a lot of other people, but George wondered if they actually had any really trustworthy friends, friends who were not just attracted by the money and power. The psychologist had also mentioned the necessity for rigorous honesty. George was not convinced that it is actually possible to live adaptively or successfully in our society and practice rigorous honesty. While George was usually an honest person, it seemed obvious that very many of the large businesses, governmental agencies, institutions, and associations in our nation often do not tell the truth. It seems that they tell whatever they want the consumer public to hear, and they almost always get away with it. That kind of action seemed to be the standard operating procedure in our society, certainly in our business dealings. But, the psychologist was suggesting something radically different than this.

The result of George's mistrust in the world, which he considered to be the *status quo* for life in the U.S., left him with a low level of anxiety, disappointment, and loneliness. But George assumed that probably everyone felt that way underneath their smiling facades. And he found that a few drinks in the evening took the edge off of life. And it was very easy to find other people to join him in that escape. They too, seemed to just want to get off the merry-go-round for a few hours, to just check-out. That seemed to be the society's approved method of softening reality, avoiding boredom, laughing a little more, and finding friends for at least a few hours. Then, in George's mind, everyone had to return to the gray reality of life. But, he told himself, at least he wasn't addicted to pills or drugs. Alcohol really worked just as well and, in George's mind, almost everyone drank alcohol. So George adopted a work-hard, play-hard philosophy, and the second edition of his addicted life began.

Perhaps the most essential thing to understand about addiction is that it is a disease-like syndrome, which can manifest through the excessive and repetitive use of various substances, behaviors, and actions in order to *alter the emotions* of the addict. The alcoholic, drug addict (any kind of drug), compulsive shopper, sex addict, compulsive gambler, compulsive overeater, true workaholic, compulsive golf addict, and addicts with many other repetitive compulsions, all have essentially the same disease.   And they often will substitute (or add) one addiction for another depending on availability. In other words, the substance or repetitive action is not the disease; it is the *symptom* of the disease.   Most addiction therapists agree that the addiction disease or syndrome is essentially the same psychologically regardless of the symptom displayed.   In addition, addictions of all kinds typically activate the same pleasure pathways in the brain. Of course, the reasons behind the choice of drug for the individual addict or the particular action repeated compulsively can be the result of a multitude of factors. Also, with time, the kind of drug or chosen addictive behavior usually will have its own particular reflexive influence on the individual. The individual often develops a bizarre neurotic relationship with the drug or behavior of choice, similar to an obsessive illicit love (hate) affair.

The disease of addiction is a problem having to do primarily with the emotions of the individual. In some ways, addicts are hypersensitive emotionally, and they do not tolerate stress well. Addiction is a disease of extremism. Consequently, the emotions of the addict are often experienced internally as extreme or excessive. For instance, relatively small or moderate stresses may be experienced as major crises for the addict. In the opposite direction, small or moderate pleasures may be rated as almost ecstatic. The emotions of the addict are labile and easily change or switch from one extreme to another. The very *intensity* of emotions for the addict provides a sort of heightened meaning, hence *bliss in a bottle.* The actual effect of the drug or alcohol on the addict is typically more intense than for the normal person. Therefore, for someone like George, who has not found much meaning in his life, the altered emotions brought on by alcohol or drugs provide a seemingly easy escape from reality, a way to accentuate certain feelings and dampen others.

Addiction, contrary to the opinion of most ordinary people, is a disease of control. The addict may appear *out* of control by conventional standards, but he or she has *chosen* to alter his or her reality in a particular direction. That direction is perceived as a better (easier, softer, more exciting, less stressful, etc.) way of being than straight reality. Escape from everyday life is typically the goal. The addict is not willing to live life on *life's* terms. However, as in George's case, the addict's perception of the everyday state of reality is skewed or distorted. Usually, the addict's view of life is too limited. She or he does not trust that the 'happiness' others talk about in their lives is really possible or attainable for him/herself. Distrust of others and of the world in general is common among addicts. The addict sees him/herself as 'different'. Addicts almost all suffer from a distorted view of themselves, feeling essential shame and lack of self worth. The well known arrogance of alcoholics is actually a cover for the basic lack of self worth or feelings of inferiority. Interpersonally, addicts tend to withdraw from true intimacy, because they are afraid of the rigorous honesty necessary for close relationship. Addicts eventually live lives full of pretense, because they do not trust that they can be real with anyone, not even themselves.

All of these factors, taken together, produce an individual who does not trust many aspects of reality that are commonly accepted by the average person. He or she feels stuck in a life which is not tolerable, but does not trust that the life touted by healthy folks can be real. Part of this dilemma is that eventually the addict does not believe that real and consistent honesty exists anywhere. And, in a society where dishonesty is commonplace, even at the highest echelons of government, the health industry, and big business, there seems to be little to support a standard of truthfulness. Unfortunately, our society at large acts as an addict, and teaches addiction to its citizens. In those cases where an individual has not grown up in a supportive and predictable environment, or has been abused by those who should love her/him, or has not received the appropriate social education, avoiding addiction can be especially difficult. In order to overcome or recover from addiction and to get real mental health, individuals must, in many ways, go against the grain of our addictive culture. To be mentally healthy, people must rise above the low standards of our corrupt society.

To be clear, addiction has its roots in an untrue, distorted, and limited view of reality. Taken all together, the addictions are probably the most prevalent health problem in the U.S. This is not surprising, in view of the fact that the society as a whole is an addict. For sure, there are no societies without some level of addiction. However, ours is one of the sickest, because it is one of the richest materially and financially, but is among the poorest in terms of covert manipulations, dishonesty, misleading advertising, and outright greed. We Americans are masters at creating false images. Like all other addicts, our society wants others to believe the image we show them, not the real truth of the situation. Bait-and-switch is a very American game; we could have invented it.

Persons with addictions often have low self-esteem, feel anxious if they do not have control over their environment, and they often come from psychologically and/or physically abusive families. However, addiction is considered by most addiction specialists to be a *primary* disorder. In other words, the addiction is a disease unto itself; it is not just the symptom of another problem. There is no consensus or agreement among addiction specialists as to the causes of addiction. However, there is clarity about the essential characteristics of addiction: Addictions are *chronic* as opposed to acute. Acute (short term) diseases can be cured; chronic (long term) diseases cannot be cured, only managed. Most addictions are *progressive.* That is, they tend to get worse over time. And addictions are most often *incurable*, especially the substance addictions, but also many behavioral addictions. As a result, the addict will never be able to *safely* use the substance again, and the behavioral addict (process addict) may never be able to *safely* go into environments associated with his or her addiction (recovering gamblers cannot safely go into casinos, etc.).

Some of the common psychological defense mechanisms used by addicts include denial, projection, rationalization, intellectualization, and several others. The addict usually *denies* to her/himself and others that there is actually a problem. This is a refusal to accept the truth, as it is pointed out by others. The addict often *projects* the responsibility for her/his problems onto other people, particularly those who criticize him/her. The addict, in effect, says, "I don't have a problem; *you* simply have a problem with me". Addicts often try to *rationalize* their addictive behaviors. This is an attempt to make the behavior sound like a logical consequence of the life situation in which the addict finds him/herself. This is the point at which the addict typically reasons to her/himself and to others, that the drug, alcohol, or addictive behavior is the result of anxiety, depression, stress, or other life problems. The addict's attempt to rationalize the addictive behavior is the primary reason that most non-addicts believe that addiction is the result of some other problem. It is not. There may be *acute* abuses of drugs, alcohol, or other compulsive behaviors by almost anyone, which seem to be a reaction to short-term stresses in a person's life. However, these periods of acute compulsive use are transient, and they cease after a relatively short period. The addict, however, does not stop; the substance or behavior abuse continues until the addiction takes on a life of its own. At this point, there is no reasonable explanation for its continuity. Addicts are also likely to try to *intellectualize* their addictions. Intellectualizing is similar to rationalizing; it is an attempt to provide some reason, ranging from mundane to philosophical, for the addictive behavior. It is an attempt on the addict's part to distance him/herself from the feelings of pain, misery, guilt, and shame associated with the addictive behavior.

Addiction is said to be a *primary* disorder. However, in the case of addiction, there *is* a causal factor with which it is always associated. It is an existential factor; that is, it has to do with what life is and what life means. As mentioned previously, the addict does not accept life on life's terms; she or he maintains a distorted view of reality in general. As in most mental illnesses, the amount of distortion can range from a little to a lot. The distortions can range from paranoid conspiracy theories, to virtually complete lack of trust in self or others, to distortions of scientific facts about the world, to a very warped view of interpersonal relationships, to a multitude of other incorrect pieces of information and misunderstandings of basic reality. In the worst cases, addicts can be actively hallucinating psychotics; in the mildest cases the distortions can seem almost reasonable to the average person. Addiction has virtually no correlation with intelligence. Some addicts are extremely intelligent and/or talented, and their intellectual prowess may even work against them, because they often are more aware and can see clearly the amount of dishonesty in the society. This is the reason that truth is perhaps the single most important factor in mental health, and for avoiding and treating addictions.

4

MEDICAL VERSUS PSYCHOLOGICAL

It all began with Sigmund Freud, or at least we can use his psychoanalytic theory as a convenient reference point. Freud was an Austrian neurologist who was one of the first to use talk therapy as a treatment for psychological problems. In this sense, he was the first psychotherapist who used treatments similar to those used today by psychologists, some psychiatrists, counselors, and mental health specialists who treat mental problems. As a physician in the early 1900s, he was very motivated to see his method, which he called 'psychoanalysis', accepted as a legitimate scientific method of treatment. Also, clinical psychology and psychiatry were in their infancy, and wanted to be accepted into the scientific community, along with physics, chemistry, biology, etc. However, these other accepted fields of science were *physical* sciences, based on the philosophy of science called *logical positivism*. This philosophy is very appropriate for dealing with the *material* and physical aspects of reality. This philosophy of science professes that *reductionism,* the practice of subdividing phenomena into pieces, and seeing how the pieces fit together, is the way science should be conducted. But psychology, the science of mind, generally would not, in reality, conform to that method of exploration. Nevertheless, Freud was, first a medical doctor, and second a brain doctor. His training had most definitely been in dealing with the physical aspects of reality. Therefore, he assumed that the mind was essentially the brain in action. He believed that science would eventually discover that all the characteristics we consider to be aspects of the mind are actually complex functions of the brain.[15]

Modern psychiatry was born out of Freud's original thinking, and it became a specialty in *medicine.* Freud was extremely popular, and the field of medicine was more than willing to accept him and the new field of psychiatry into its fold. The first psychoanalysts (those therapists who practiced Freud's method) were virtually all medical doctors, and so, a new medical specialty was born.

The inherent difficulty in considering all mental difficulties to be only brain problems is obvious. That argument simply does not hold up to scrutiny. The mind, and so many aspects of human behavior, beliefs, aspirations, relationships, and life meaningfulness, are simply larger than just the brain alone. Brain alone cannot account for the huge impact of beliefs, values, courage, determination, compassion, life meaning, and consciousness itself. Mind is one of those phenomena for which the whole is much greater than the sum of the parts we can name, let alone measure. It is a holistic entity, in some ways a mirror for all aspects of life (more about mind vs. brain in later chapters).

Psychology is one of the youngest of the major fields of science. Although it seems obvious that the study of the mind, in general, belongs in the science of psychology, brain function is a significant factor in some parts of the functioning of the mind. This may suggest, at first glance, that psychiatry is right in its assumption that mind is brain function. However, this is an antiquated conceptualization of the mind. Nevertheless, the formal, organized medical sciences (physical sciences) are much older than the younger science of psychology; which means that the medical sciences have deeper roots in the culture and tradition of healing. And, the necessity for physical treatment is often an immediate critical priority on the list of needs for wellbeing, while the treatment of psychological issues is often not an emergency need; and the treatment often takes longer. Physical symptoms can be seen or sensed physically in the observable world, or at least with the physical senses. Mind symptoms, involving thinking and feeling and relationships are often much more subtle, often obscure or not so obvious to the physical observer. Another very significant reason for the tendency of people to think of psychiatry as more important than psychology is the gigantic political power of the American Medical Association (A.M.A.). In spite of the flawed scientific practices and incorrect philosophy of science used by psychiatry, organized medicine has been able to market psychiatrists as the gate keepers of mental health. Psychiatry has, in effect, been able to hide behind the skirts of the A.M.A.

In today's world, professional mental health care has evolved into two main camps, the medical, represented by the field of psychiatry, and the psychological, represented primarily by the broad field of clinical psychology. Psychiatrists have medical degrees and their primary training is in physical medicine. They have more extensive training in brain function and physiology than psychologists do. Psychologists have doctor's degrees in psychology and their primary training is in the study of the mind. They have more extensive training in psychology and mental diagnosis than psychiatrists. A benefit of this division of labor is that the medical doctors are primarily in charge of administering drug therapy, while the psychologists are primarily in charge of psycho-diagnostics and psychotherapy. Typically psychiatrists do not do psychotherapy, and psychologists do not prescribe drugs. In the optimal situation there is collusion and communication between the two for the benefit of the patient. In support of this joint effort, research into the treatment of many kinds of *serious* mental health problems shows that the optimal treatment program is often a combination of psychotherapy and drugs. Nevertheless, the treatment of a large proportion of the problems brought to psychologists and psychiatrists do not need the additional brain alteration provided by psychoactive medications for optimal healing to occur. For these patients, usually those with less severe symptoms, drugs often only confuse the issues by masking the symptoms temporarily. Also, drugs often reduce the patient's motivation to obtain psychotherapy to deal with the real causes. But a patient is almost certain to obtain drugs for his or her difficulties, large or small, if he or she happens to see a psychiatrist first without consulting some other mental health consultant beforehand. In other words, the psychiatrist sees through the eyes of what is called the *medical model*, and assumes that all psychological complaints are physical in origin. She or he treats patients the way every physician has been taught to treat patients, physically. However, *psychiatry has never been able to demonstrate scientifically how any chemical imbalance or chemical inconsistency in the brain causes psychological problems.*[15] It can only show that certain chemicals will alleviate some of the *symptoms* of selected mental problems at least some of the time. This is perhaps the most basic example of how the materialistic bias in our society teaches us to trade real mental health for addiction. Very many of the so-called *psychotropic* medications (the kind that psychiatrists prescribe) are potentially addictive, at least psychologically. In this case, the medical profession itself is creating and perpetuating addiction, directly and indirectly. Psychiatrists profess and perpetuate the idea that medications are actually a *cure* for mental illness. That is not the truth. The very profession that should be one of the main standard bearers of mental health is duping its own patients and teaching addiction, wittingly or unwittingly. There are, of course, a minority of fine, discriminating psychiatrists who recognize the fallacy in this kind of blanket prescribing, and are prompt to recommend psychotherapy without medication in some cases. It also should be noted that most psychologists and other non-medical psychotherapists are usually not adverse to the idea of medication; but they are very cautious about recommending it. There is a clear recognition among psychologists and other mental health professionals that medication is often counterproductive to the ultimate resolution of problems, and should not be recommended in most cases.

George felt that he was functioning fairly well. He continued to use alcohol to ameliorate his boredom and unrest, and it seemed to do the trick most of the time. He did notice, however, that he was beginning to slowly increase the amount he consumed. It seemed to take a little more alcohol to soothe his soul as time went on. George maintained the rhythms of his life, sometimes rigidly, and was often displeased when his schedule got upset or changed unexpectedly. He avoided events and venues where alcohol was not available. The importance of alcohol took on more and more meaning in George's life. He began to withdraw attention from Mary, except to fulfill his sexual needs, and she seemed unhappy and distant a lot of the time. But George, without realizing it, was really in love with the bottle, and actually, nothing else meant very much to him. People at work seemed less available for interaction with George. At first he assumed they were just busier than usual, but after a while he began to see them as not interested in him like they had been before. The boredom at work felt worse than ever. George was thankful that he could at least turn off the tedium when he got away and could drink. One day he decided that the simple solution was to take a flask with him to work. He could take a 'break' and get a few sips out of his flask in the restroom. No one would be the wiser, and that would help take the pressure off his nerves.

Fortunately for George, one day the fellow employee whom he had considered his closest work associate told George that rumors were beginning to spread about his alcohol use. He reported to George that others could smell the alcohol on his breath, and that George's behavior seemed to be different than it used to be. This was a fortunate encounter for George because it shocked him into a higher state of self-awareness, at least temporarily. George could not deny the accuracy of his associate's statements, so he responded with a simple 'thanks' to his associate and left the room. However, inside of George, his anxiety was going through the roof. He recognized that he had narrowly avoided real trouble with his employer.

George, having talked to a psychologist before, recognized the value of having a safe, confidential place to process his problems with someone who could at least mirror back to him the sound and feel of his own statements. And George knew, from that earlier experience, that whatever decisions or changes were to be made would be his own; the psychotherapist was simply George's consultant, and was bound legally to keep George's information confidential. George also knew that prescription drugs were not the answer to his problems. He had tried that before with the psychiatrist. He was so thankful that he was no longer a 'drug' addict. George assumed that alcohol is not really a drug in the same way that other psychoactive substances are. After all, it is legal and is used by very many people in our society. Use of alcohol is traditional; how can it be a big problem? Alcohol did not seem to be dangerous like real drugs, unless a person is an alcoholic. George certainly didn't consider himself to be an alcoholic. He reasoned that he had simply been indiscrete. He needed to be more careful. Nevertheless, he wished he could talk to someone about his life. He still really was not happy. He had the sense that he was just treading water in his life. Surely there had to be something better than this. He just couldn't discover what it is. So, George decided to go back to the psychologist, and to try to approach his problems from a different direction than he had before. He somehow had to find out what was *missing* in his life. He wondered, fleetingly, if the psychologist may actually have been right before, when he talked about that ideal of real happiness, which seemed like an unattainable dream. He would make another appointment with the psychologist and re-explore.

The essential argument between psychology and psychiatry is the difference between the psychological conceptualization of *mind* and the medical psychiatric *presumption* that mind is only brain. Materialism is again the culprit. Psychiatry's science attempts to reduce reality to the smallest pieces possible, *things*. It bases this tactic on a scientific tradition which was

designed for dealing with the manifest physical world. In
order to be accepted (back in Freud's era) as one of the
physical sciences, psychiatry simply decided to treat all mental
issues from a physical point of view. Psychiatry continues to
adhere to this tradition, in spite of the fact that this is
antiquated thinking with no actual scientific basis. Legitimate
modern science, in virtually every other field of inquiry, has
moved far beyond the antiquated thinking of psychiatry. Even
most branches of biology and physiology have moved on to
recognize that other kinds of research derived from a more
sophisticated philosophy are necessary to describe the
livingness that is the essence of life. The aliveness of humans,
the vital force, is a process, not a thing; and it must be
considered and treated from a holistic point of view.

Modern psychotherapy, or mental health counseling, is of
course talk therapy, but it has moved far past Freud's original
psychoanalysis technique. Psychotherapy, in general, involves
an interactive process between a therapist and a client. While
a complete explanation of psychotherapy is beyond the scope
of this book, there are a few general theories, approaches, and
issues worth examining. First of all, it is important to realize
that psychotherapy necessitates a collusion between therapist
and client to help the client learn more about him or her self, to
undo the symptoms or help the client learn more positive
habits, to discover personal talents and limitations, to clarify
goals and aspirations, to explore personal history which may
be relevant to the client's problems, to restore or repair the self
image, to help the client learn to be self-confident, to help the
client discover and create life-meaning, to gain a sense of
balance in life, to deal constructively with relationships, and
hopefully to be happy. Although this may seem like a huge
task, it is the work of life. It primarily is to help a person
examine him/herself with love and objectivity, as well as
subjectively and emotionally. Some types of therapy focus on
short-term problem resolution without in-depth examination
of the client's life. However, even those short-term therapies

must consider the long term results. All problems exist within a system of other factors, which help maintain and perpetuate the problem. Otherwise, the problem behaviors would cease for lack of acceptance or reinforcement from others. And all persons exist in a system of other people who influence and encourage them, directly or indirectly, to maintain or change the personal image they portray to others. Therefore, virtually all problems of living have to do, directly or indirectly, with relationships with other people. 'No man is an island', as the saying goes. Consequently, the kinds of issues which get dealt with in psychotherapy and counseling can range from minute bad habits, such as obsessive finger tapping, to huge existential and philosophical meaning-of-life issues, and virtually everything in between. Psychotherapy treats symptoms and causes. Treatment with psychotherapy works because, hopefully, it goes directly to the heart, and science, and philosophy of how to live an adaptive, happy, and productive life in our society. As the old saying goes, 'people are all the same, and people are all different'. Therefore, one of the main goals of counseling and psychotherapy is to help a person accept and honor his or her uniqueness; and another goal is to help the client live in happy relationship with others, and to honor her/his similarities to others. Psychotherapy, like life itself, must be grounded in science, logic, good judgment, and rigorous honesty. However the other side of psychotherapy, like life itself, must be grounded in intuition, life as art, emotion, personal values, and passion for life. Ultimately, only the balance and mix of these two, science and art (or intellect and emotion), can result in the kind of happiness and life-fulfillment which is rounded and complete.

5

BRAIN VERSUS MIND

In the year 1641 the French philosopher Rene Descartes
declared, "I think, therefore I am." With that statement, he
began a new system of physical science, which included only
those things that could be detected directly by the five human
physical senses.[16] Descartes' statement reasserted a dualistic
view of body and mind, much like Plato and Aristotle before
him. This view states that mind and body are separate entities.
It asserts that some intellectual mechanisms are located in the
brain, but mind itself is a separate function, not directly related
to the body. This dualistic view is still today the prevalent
belief of most people in our society. Most people agree that
such concepts as motivations, attitudes, values, compassion,
altruism, and belief in truth, for example, cannot possibly be
reduced only to the actions of brain cells.

Descartes' famous statement also pointed to that aspect of
mind we now call *consciousness*. Consciousness is that aspect
of mind which allows us to sense ourselves *subjectively* in the
present moment, and also allows us to seemingly stand outside
ourselves and look back *objectively*, to intellectualize about
ourselves as autonomous creatures among other creatures and
objects. The study of consciousness has become a major
cutting-edge concern in science. For instance, modern
research in quantum physics must, of necessity, consider the
role of the *experimenter* along with the roles of the other
factors in any experiment.[17] The *wishes* of the experimenter
exert their own influence on the outcome of experiments.
Strange as this may seem, it is the nature of the quantum
world. For example, a light beam can be measured and
recorded as either light waves or particles (photons). If the
experimenter wishes to measure particles, the result of his or
her demonstration will be particles; but if the experimenter
wishes to measure waves, the result will show waves. It is
totally dependent on which quality of nature the experimenter

intends to see. Therefore, modern science has discovered the seminal importance of studying the effects of consciousness itself. In fact, Leonard Susskind, the astrophysicist whose theory of black holes has currently replaced Stephen Hawking's theory,[18] as the leading comprehensive theory-of–almost-everything, concludes that time, space, matter, and virtually everything else we consider everyday reality, are actually *secondary*, illusory aspects of some underlying *unitary*, or undivided reality. Susskind and his associates propose that ultimate reality is somewhat like a hologram; and each individual is like a piece of the holograph, reflecting and projecting the image of the whole. In other words, each of us is like a mirror reflecting the image of all of the other individual mirrors and the image of the whole of reality all at once. But ultimately, the primary aspect of reality is the whole. In this sense everything is, and we are, all one thing. Mind bending as it seems, material reality is at least partly the result of our *intention* to perceive it. It is our *consciousness.* [17] Other findings which support the quantum physicists' conclusions that time, space, and matter are malleable and relative comes from the study of parapsychology (the study of so-called *psychic* phenomena). Dean Radin, the brilliant senior researcher at the Center For Noetic Sciences, reviewed, critiqued, threw out flawed studies, and eventually did massive meta-analyses of more than a thousand controlled studies of extrasensory experience over the last century.[19] The analysis of these studies demonstrates, with combined odds against chance of more than 10^{104} to 1, that some psychic phenomena really do exist. This research demonstrates, beyond the shadow of a doubt, that we humans somehow have connections to other persons and things which are beyond the limits of reason, and beyond the limits of time, space, and matter. So, what does all of this mean, and what does it have to do with addiction, mental health, and truth? For one thing, it means that the argument about whether mind is more than just brain is completely settled. It means essentially that *mind is everything.* No thing exists outside of our consciousness.

Descartes' mind-body dualism has been undone by the advance of the scientific regime which he (and a few others) started.

Questions about consciousness, mind, intention, and awareness all point to one essential question, 'what is the life force itself?' In addition to the findings of quantum physics, the science of biology has discovered some interesting things about the life force and about mind. Living organisms at all levels seem to exist in a huge context of other living things. The autonomy of individual organisms is in essence an illusion. There are many levels of organization of life, and living forms almost always exist in colonial clusters, which are intertwined and enfolded in one another. The human body, for instance, consists of billions of different organisms. It has been said that the number of distinctly human cells in the human body is approximately only one tenth of the total number of all living cells in the body.[20] Our bodies consist of colonies of cells of other living organisms including bacteria, viruses, and others which have no definite classification. And we are apparently dependent on virtually all of them for the balanced functioning of our bodies. Each of us humans is, therefore, a huge mega-colony of various living creatures.

This intertwined, symbiotic, colonial pattern is very common in nature, essentially the norm for all living things. It even calls into question the way we traditionally conceptualize our intelligence (mind). For example, there are some species of sea sponges which can be shredded into their individual living cells without killing the cells in the process. When these individual living cells are left in fresh flowing sea water, after several hours they will rejoin themselves into the *exact* same sponge which was shredded in the first place, down to the fine details.[21] And sponges have no nervous system, no brain, and every sponge is unique in shape. Modern biology demonstrates that this organizing intelligence of life operates not just within the cell, not just within the single complex organism, and not just within the colony, but even between species. Viewed in this way, the boundaries between various living things appear vague, indefinite, and complex. We are immersed and enmeshed in many systems of life; and we are autonomous in only a relative way. Truly, no person is an island. Ultimately, all of life is connected in a dancing, ever-moving, and ever-changing web of energy. Mind at large, or vital force, or spirit of life, or ultimate reality is the overarching mind of life, which is beneath, within, between and beyond all things. These facts are state-of-the-art, cutting edge knowledge revealed by the sciences which describe life processes. It seems that our lives are mediated and controlled by some overarching field of consciousness, some ubiquitous energy field, which is comparable to what the world's great spiritual traditions have called God. It should be noted that humans have never been able to create the life force. In spite of the apparent sophistication of science to add, subtract, multiply, and divide living tissue and matter, it has never been able to give life to physical matter that was not already alive. Life itself is that thing which is beyond our capacity to grasp.

Cosmology and theoretical physics have proposed theories of ultimate reality such as the hologram (mentioned above), parallel universes, string theories, the multiverse, etc.[22] But, whether we describe ultimate reality in cosmic terms such as these, they are theories which are beyond the capacity of humans to actually prove. They cannot actually be proved because, if they do exist as anything more than mathematical deductions, they exist beyond the level of the five human senses. Further, if they could be proved, they are explanations of some ultimate organization of reality far beyond time, space, and person and they offer no new insight to humans. What they do offer is consensual validation for the view that ultimate reality is *spiritual* in quality, beyond space, time, and person, yet ever present. In view of the fact that we cannot and will not actually comprehend these things in any foreseeable future, they *do not* offer an improved explanation of ultimate reality. For practical purposes they only offer substitutes for the word God. God is, by definition, that concept which is beyond the limits of accurate or total description, essentially the same as the explanation above offered by science. It appears that science has come full circle, and must now admit that humans' intuitive awareness of some higher, transcendent power has been correct, natural, and instinctive all along. The concept is the same; it is that ultimate thing or force which has no discernable boundaries, no limits, and cannot be grasped with the human mind. It is totally mystical.

This new wave of science has also prompted psychology, especially clinical psychology, to re-examine itself and focus on those issues having to do with holism and the study of consciousness. In particular, it necessitates moving away from explanations having to do with the material *content* of life. It must focus more on the relational *process* issues of life. In other words, the attention of mental health specialists should be focused not on material *brain* issues, but on holistic *living* issues. Classical Newtonian physics (everyday physics), as an explanation for how the whole of life works, is insufficient. It only explains how that part of life which is secondary and illusory works. The correct (in so far as we are able to describe it with words) explanation for real life is in the processes of consciousness, a holistic view of what is most important, relationships, connections, and communications. We cannot escape material reality and remain conscious, but we can live in constant awareness that the material world is an illusion. Life is inherently mystical. It seems important to note that most wisdom traditions, including virtually all the great spiritual traditions, have been recommending for millennia that the best way to live is not to focus on the material, but on the ethereal aspects of life; not the things, but the relationships among people, not the content, but the processes of life.

As a result of our new scientific reframing of reality, we must learn to think a new way. We find that even our language (especially the language of the Western world) is not oriented correctly for thinking the new way. English, as one of the Germanic languages, is a content oriented language. But the new paradigm for reality focuses on a flowing, ever changing, relational world. It needs process oriented language. Some of the aboriginal languages seem to capture it best, because they are based on a mystical view of life.[23] The basic precepts of our English language must eventually change. Also, we are on the precipice of a shift in the way science conducts itself and how it conducts research. There are still a significant number of scientists who will not accept that reality acts in such irrational ways as noted above. More and more of these staid traditional scientists, however, are realizing that they will be left behind like the farmer plowing with the aid of a mule instead of a tractor if they do not change. Science and spirituality have come to a meeting of the minds as never before in history. New has come full circle to meet old, in essential agreement for the first time. The *objective* rational approach of science, having pursued ultimate reality to the limits of its own descriptive abilities, has found itself in essential agreement with the basic *subjectively* revealed truths of religion (not the specific dogma of any one religion).

The implications of the new paradigm suggest, not that we try to forgo the material world and live on some different plane of existence (at least not completely), but that we wear the world like a loose garment. Living in the new paradigm implies that we should try to raise our consciousness to a new level of awareness. We should try to live with the constant awareness that we are connected to each other and to all of reality in a very essential way; we truly are all *the same being.*

George explained to the psychotherapist his seeming dilemma; he understood that the therapist had been alluding to some peaceful existence, based in truth, which does not need medication to feel right and happy. But, George told the therapist that he had become aware that he didn't really trust most people to actually tell the truth, and certainly not governments, big business, or institutions. Consequently, it was difficult for George to believe that living transparently and responsibly could result in his being happy. After all, he reasoned, if he was living with lies all around him, how could he protect himself by being rigorously honest while everyone else (in George's eyes) is cheating. Seeing his client's sincere wish to find real life meaning, the psychologist began to explain to George the latest research of science in physics, biology, psychology, and parapsychology, and about the need to include consciousness itself as the essential ingredient. He suggested to George that real meaning exists not in the mundane world of things; but that life-at-large beyond time, space, and matter is the current state of knowledge about ultimate reality. The therapist also alluded to the fact that this larger truth of life from science fits most religious and spiritual traditions' concept of a God. The therapist was careful to explain that he was not talking about religion *per se,* but the idea of spirituality in general.

George's first response was to look at the therapist skeptically and wonder if he had encountered some New-Age snake oil salesman, who was suggesting that George pretend that reality doesn't exist. However, he trusted the therapist because of their contract with each other. The therapist reminded George often that any decisions were George's to make for himself; the therapist was just his consultant. The psychologist explained further that the idea is not to forsake the everyday material reality we know, but to constantly be aware that it is illusory, transient, relative, and not to be trusted to provide real life meaning and happiness. Real meaning, said the therapist, is to be found in the relationships between people, in the creative processes which arise from emotion, and a reverence for all of life which transcends everyday things. Wear the everyday world like a loose garment; it is not the true essence of life.

These ideas, in the beginning, were so mind-blowing for George that he felt disoriented and insecure, as if he was in limbo between heaven and hell. He was both very excited and also anxious. What he now understood with his rational mind is that what he *thought* he knew rationally before was not actual truth. How could one live with his or her feet in two separate worlds at the same time? George began to research the scientific issues on the internet, and then in books. He came to thoroughly understand the conclusions of the research findings. These findings had been unfolding gradually for decades; they were supported by a majority of the most prominent and the most brilliant scientists in the world. The experiments had been repeated over and over hundreds of times with the same results. He felt a real sense of excitement that he had not felt in a long time, maybe never. He wanted to share his new-found knowledge with others, but he was afraid that if he tried, he would be rejected as a lunatic by most of the people he knew. George had lost his interest in escaping from reality with alcohol almost completely. He simply felt no urge to drink like before. He had become more pleasant and constructive in his interactions with fellow workers and with Mary. One day, George's friend who had warned him in the past about his indiscretions with alcohol at work, mentioned how nice it was to see a happier George. George felt moved to share with his friend what had happened to him. To George's amazement, his friend reported that he also had recovered from alcoholism and drug addiction some years ago, and had come to essentially the same conclusions about reality. George asked him how he had managed to stop using alcohol and drugs and be happy. The friend told George he attended Alcoholics Anonymous meetings, and found many other people there who believed in a reality similar to George's. He said he also had friends who attended other kinds of meetings and self-help groups, even some in certain churches which are involved in recovery from addictions and other mental health problems. His friend said that his group provided a forum of other people to share with, whose experiences and beliefs were, in many ways, similar to his own. He went to a meeting with his friend, and George did in fact find others who could appreciate his own experience and knowledge. The support of the group and of the individuals there helped George to feel like he belonged, and it gave him consensual validation for his beliefs. He continued to see the psychologist off and on for some time, realizing the benefit of having a consultant to process life's occasional stresses. Within a few months, George realized that he was happy in a way that he did not know is possible until he had tried it for a while. Almost every day seemed to offer George new opportunities to interact with other people in some constructive way, some way to make someone else feel better or to make them laugh. The paradoxical thing was that George himself seemed to be the big winner as a result of his care for others. He really was beginning to understand that we and all of reality are *all one being.*

6

TRADING MENTAL HEALTH FOR ADDICTION

In the Latin writings of Marcus Aurelius Antoninus (121-180
A.D.), the great general, philosopher, and Caeser of Rome (161-
180 A.D.), he stated, *"Espiritum vinci espiritus"*---Higher power
(spirit) overcomes alcoholism (the effects of spirits of alcohol).
The great Swiss psychiatrist Carl Jung (1875-1961) pointed out
these same words in his treatment of an alcoholic in 1930, who
was able to use this information to recover from his severe
alcoholism.[24] This prescription was passed on to Bill Wilson,
the founder of Alcoholics Anonymous. The idea became the
central theme of Alcoholics Anonymous, which has become the
prime standard for treatment of alcoholism the world over.[25]
A more modern version of the above is, *every addict is seeking
mystical or spiritual experience.*

Most of our population seems not to recognize the importance
of the ideas in the paragraph above. These ideas point out the
disbelief of the typical alcoholic such as George, and the power
of the necessary shift in consciousness, from seeing the world
in mundane, materialistic terms to seeing the world as sacred
and transcendent. The addict whose addiction has progressed
over time loses his or her way in a maze of distortions of
perception, and no longer measures reality correctly. Memory
abilities are dampened and distorted and judgment impaired.
Even during periods of seeming clear-headedness, when the
effects of the drug have worn off after sleep, the attitude of the
addict is fatalistic at least, and suicidal at worst. The belief in
the value and meaning of life has been lost or so warped as to
be destructive in a myriad of ways. The only viable way out of
this downward spiral is to find a new vision of life that is
imbued with new meaning. A huge number of people in our
society live in a sort of fatalistic limbo with no real sense of
meaning for their lives. The sad fact is that these are the
citizens who are most vulnerable to the lure of addictions sold
and/or supported by the pharmaceutical companies, the

twisted health system, and corrupt politicians. They are at high risk of becoming willing victims of the very systems which profess to be helping and healing them. And once they are caught in the whirlwind, it can be very difficult to recover.

Contrast the vicious circle of addiction with its polar opposite, high-level mental health. Mental health, seen through the eyes of the new perspective, goes beyond the limits of the mind-body argument, and points to a dynamic moving and flowing reality which is always new and always the same. While we must live in the material world, we *must* adopt a broader appreciation of life's intricate and virtually infinite interfolding of all species with one another, and with all things. What we come to realize, when we consider the cutting edge revelations of all the major sciences together, is that the life force pervades all of reality. There is a theory called the Gaia hypothesis, which points out that the earth itself actually fulfills all of the criteria for being a living organism.[26] Also, the universe fulfills all of the criteria for being a living system. While we can observe and construe the phenomena of life in terms of the physical or the mental, the underlying fabric of all of reality is spiritual (not necessarily *religious* in the traditional sense, but connoting *mystical*). What is needed is a generic word which carries the general idea of *spirit,* and carries the idea of an over-aching being, transcendent, transpersonal, trans-spatial, trans-temporal, and pervasive. The notion is to catch the meaning of the whole of reality as one living entity; that every single aspect of the conscious mind and the sensate world is a reflection of spirit-at-large.

Living life based on this knowledge necessitates a certain set of principles for thinking and acting. It implies that we should see all of life as sacred, and treat it with reverence. It implies that we should have great tolerance for differences between us, because we all are parts of the one being, attached in the same way that waves are attached to the ocean. It implies that we should always try to do the most constructive thing possible, even though we sometimes may have to choose what seems to be the lesser of two evils. It also implies that we should remember that all *things* are transient and temporary, but the *Whole of Life* remains permanent. These laws of life for humans are concordant with virtually all of the rules for living (commandments) for each of the world's great spiritual traditions, because they are essentially all the same. What is new is that now both the sacred (religion) and the secular (science) understand reality essentially the same way. Every single thing in the universe, from the smallest to the largest, is alive and sacred. The results of this thinking and pattern for living are not only true happiness, but high level mental health. The person who utilizes these principles for living is much more resistant to the lures and traps of addiction perpetuated by the dishonesty and destruction done by big business, the health industry, and corrupt politicians.

Whether a person becomes a serious student of the new science, in order to avoid or escape the tentacles of addiction in our culture there must be an appreciation of some kind of ultimate meaning and value for life. Otherwise, the fate of a growing proportion of our population, and consequently a growing threat to the whole nation, is at stake. The new science offers, even to those who are not religiously oriented, a new life philosophy based on the findings of research. Those without direction or purpose can no longer rationalize away their apathy as distrust in religion and religious ideas. The most basic principle of virtually all religions, the belief in a higher power, who/which is basically benevolent, has now been validated with scientific research. *The new science may offer the most hopeful light on the horizon for our nation being able to reverse its progressive decline into addiction and chaos.* The basic transcendent truth, which has been intuitively revealed to the religiously oriented throughout the eons of time, has now also been revealed to the scientifically oriented through their measurements and quantifications. Science has been struck by ethereal lightning, and is as awed and mystified as the prophets of old.

7

THE COMMERCIALIZATION OF MENTAL HEALTH

Each new prescription medication which comes on the market must be shown to be effective in order for the pharmaceutical company to have it approved by the Federal Drug Administration. A certain set of experimental steps must be carried out. These steps are the *research standards* acceptable to the scientific community. One of the standards of proof is the necessity to repeat the same experiment on another group of patients and get similar results. If these experimental demonstrations are successful, the drug company is then allowed to advertise the results to the public, claiming that their new drug helps in the treatment of some medical problem. However, a multitude of dishonest research practices, dishonest marketing tactics, and unscrupulous dealings with Congress on the part of some of the big pharmaceutical companies have been well documented by a number of different writers, most often by doctors themselves. In recent years, books such as **The Truth About The Drug Companies, how they deceive us and what to do about it,** by Marcia Angell, M.D.,[27] previously editor in chief of the *New England Journal of Medicine* is a scorching expose' of the shady dealings of some of the largest drug producers and marketers, and how they buy influence in Congress and the F.D.A. Also, **Unhinged, the trouble with psychiatry,** by Daniel J. Carlat, M.D.,[28] a psychiatrist himself, offers deep insight into the ways drug companies obscure research results by duping doctors into touting and marketing their drugs to other doctors, and into the ways drug companies twist research findings to make them appear much better than they actually are. **Selling Sickness,** by Ray Moynihan and Alan Cassels,[29] and **Overdosed America**, by John Abramson, M.D.,[30] offer further evidence about how many of the big drug producers and marketers corrupt science and use egregious and unscrupulous marketing practices. These authors who have written about this corruption are some of the champions in our society's critically important fight against dishonesty, deceit, and egregious parasitic destruction, which occurs at the highest echelons of industry, medicine, and government today.

Loosely conceptualized, the factions involved in the *dishonest* commercialization of mental health are three in number, although there are many other ancillary involvements. The first of the three consists of those pharmaceutical companies (big pharma) whose conduct is designed to maximize their own profits regardless of the injury to the public they proclaim to serve. Dishonesty of many forms in the service of greed is their crime. They are extremely politically active, and appear motivated almost totally by the profit incentive. The second faction is the government, generally the members of Congress and other political candidates who prostitute themselves to those who will fund their campaigns. They often make promises of favors to their benefactors upfront before they are elected, and then find themselves at the beck and call of their contributors in order to assure that they will be reelected. This crass 'government for sale' scheme is a huge thorn in the side of democracy. In the case of big pharma, who have funded countless corruptions of members of Congress, it has resulted in disastrous consequences for health, especially mental health, in the U.S. The third dishonest faction is the medical industry, and in this case, the psychiatric branch, which hangs on to its existence as a legitimate medical specialty only tenuously. It has no legitimate scientific basis for treatment of the mind, and so finds itself in collusion with big pharma to maintain the *illusion* of legitimacy. The American Medical Association, with its huge political power, is implicit in the dishonesty by providing a cover for psychiatry to hide behind. Big pharma spends humongous amounts of money to entertain and influence medical doctors to prescribe their companies' drugs; and they often offer inaccurate and/or incomplete research findings to sell doctors on their products. In other words, some drug companies actually knowingly alter and twist scientific research findings to support the illusion that their drugs are viable treatments. The fact is that many of the psychotropic medications are little or no better than placebos. The way in which these three factions collude to protect and perpetuate the dishonest activity of each other is clear. The amount of destruction, graft, deceit, and outright damage to our society as a result of their dishonest collusion is staggering. The economic drain (actually theft) is large enough to fund the government of a not-so-small third world nation. The loss of health benefits to the public is so large that it is hard to measure accurately; it involves the damage done by the marketing of *inappropriate* treatments, and also the benefits withheld by not providing *appropriate* treatments. This dishonest swap occurs in the face of the fact that the appropriate treatments are generally well known and fully available. However, the medications which actually work are often cheaper and less profitable for the big drug companies than those of questionable treatment value. Also, in 2003, when Congress added a prescription drug benefit to Medicare, big pharma used its huge financial influence with Congressmen to make it illegal for Medicare to bargain with the drug companies for the best price for drugs for senior citizens. The resulting additional cost to individual seniors (which lines the pockets of the drug companies) amounts to thousands of dollars per year for some people. This kind of graft is unconscionable. These atrocious acts are detailed extensively by the writers mentioned above.

An even more dangerous issue in the long run, hidden and implicit in the dishonesty and graft, is the shell game which induces people to focus on drugs as the *essential* remedy for mental health problems. The essential issue is not about things, but beliefs, attitudes, values, and behaviors. It is about essential life meaning. That cannot be purchased with a pill. In the psychiatric model, doctors and patients are taught to medicate the emotional *symptoms* associated with disordered lives instead of dealing with the disorder directly. It is no wonder that our culture is probably the most addictive culture on earth. It is imperative that our people begin to see the lies and deceptions created and perpetuated by big drug companies, corrupt government officials, and the medical industry. If we do not change, our society will eventually dissolve into chaos. Ultimately, the only way we can change is individually, by assuming primary responsibility for our own health. We must recognize that we live in a society which will *always* try to sell us things we do not need and even things which are dangerous and destructive. Health treatments, health products, food (even baby food), drugs of every class, almost every market related to health may be corrupted by greed, deceit, and lies in order to sell us products which may not work at all. It is sad and even sickening to realize that this is the state of commerce, government, and health in our nation. We have no choice but to learn to look out for our selves and our families cautiously.

8

THE WAR ON DRUGS

In the years 1347/1348 the bubonic plague, the so-called *black death*, took hold in Europe and eventually killed an estimated 30 -60% of the entire population. The Spanish inquisition was also at full throttle during that time. Because the actual cause of the disease was unknown at the time (infected rats infested with fleas), the inquisition felt compelled to find a cause associated with the 'wrath of God'. The general consensus of the inquisition was that God's displeasure could be attributed to non-Christians and heretics who were poisoning the purity of the Church, and so bringing forth the plague. By the year 1350 over 50,000 'heretics' were killed by the inquisition in the name of God.[31]

Not so different from the Spanish inquisition, the U.S. war on drugs is one of the most atrocious and destructive activities ever to occur in America's history. Similar to the inquisition, the war on drugs seeks a cause for a disease, but is looking in the wrong place. The war on drugs did not arise because of some devious plot to cause destruction to the U.S. Like the inquisition, it came from the application of antiquated and oversimplified thinking to a problem that is somewhat complex. We all share the blame for allowing it to happen. Some substances which are psychoactive, and generally do need some regulation by government for safety's sake, have been chosen as the villain and have been declared illegal. These drugs, when unregulated, can be very dangerous, but the drugs *per se* are not the real problem. The real problem is *addiction*. Consider, for example, what is probably the most prevalent addiction in the U.S., which, like addiction to drugs, can have devastating consequences. It is called codependency. It is a true addiction. One form is a pathological addiction to 'love' relationships, and it excites the same neural pleasure pathways in the brain as drugs. It truly is a pathological addiction to people. This disease (it fulfills all of the criteria for being a disease syndrome) runs rampant in our society. Is the problem other *people*? Should we make other people illegal? That would, of course, be ludicrous, because we realize that the other people are not the problem. The problem is in the way that the addict *relates* to other people, not the people themselves. The focus of treatment must be on the disease syndrome. Exactly the same is true of drug addiction; the cause is not the drug itself, but the addict's relationship to the drug. We have been distracted by the fact that many drugs are psychoactive, and we fear their effects. Psychoactive drugs have been used throughout history, and addictions have also been common throughout history. It should be pointed out that, contrary to the belief of some people, no substance has ever been discovered which automatically induces addiction with just one use, or even with several uses. Typically, some small number of users may become addicted after only a few trials of any drug, while the vast majority of users will not become addicted.[32] The problem is not with the substance itself, but in the user's psychological and physiological makeup and the user's interaction with the drug.

In view of the thousands of lives lost each year, the gigantic financial costs to taxpayers, the creation and perpetuation of criminal enterprises, and the huge number of ruined lives of those incarcerated for what is actually a disease, not a criminal activity, the war on drugs is, indeed, an inquisition imposed on the citizens of our country.[33] The rationale has been that, even with the side effects of death and criminality and destruction, we must continue, because this is seen as a war against *criminals*; and our police mentality fears that the criminals will take over if we stop. However, there would be very few drug criminals, as such, if drugs were legalized and regulated instead of criminalized. The factions involved, primarily the federal and state governments, and the industries created to fight the war on drugs (state and federal police units assigned to drug activities, the penal industry, and others) are perpetuating what has ended up being a parasitic attack on the rest of the population.[34] Although the destruction is not intended, the war on drugs actually *creates* addiction instead of eradicating it. It creates addiction by teaching people to focus on the wrong thing, which is the essence of the addiction problem to begin with. In the face of overwhelming evidence that it does not work, how this outrageous *war on ourselves* manages to continue is difficult to comprehend.

Like the inquisition of old, the authorities and factions who support the war on drugs are using the drugs as the 'devil,' in order to avoid dealing with the real problem. And they are doing it in order to sustain an industry which is dependent on there being a war on drugs. Not only have psychoactive substances been used throughout history, but addiction is, in and of itself, a natural potential of the human mind and body. Drug usage is closely related to the innate human quest for spiritual/mystical experience.[32] As a matter of fact, psychoactive drugs have been used in various religious ceremonies (including Christian and Jewish ceremonies) as long as we have recorded history. However, *pathological* drug abuse is essentially a *substitute* for mystical/spiritual experience, which some people believe is otherwise unattainable. Addiction is the result of this substitute activity becoming a habit, which captures its victims in a lock-hold, which can be very difficult to break. But treatment and recovery is attainable; and we are gaining more insight into the causes and effective treatments for addictions at an accelerating rate.

Some statistics related to the war on drugs and its consequences:[35] The U.S. federal government spent over $15 billion dollars in 2010 on the war on drugs, at a rate of about $500 per second. State and local governments spent at least another $25 billion dollars. Arrests for drug violations for year 2012 are expected to exceed the 1,663,582 arrests of 2009. Law enforcement made more arrests for drug abuse violations (an estimated 1.6 million arrests, or 13.0 percent of the total number of arrests) than any other offense in 2009. Since 1995, the U.S. prison population has grown an average of 43,266 inmates per year. About 25 percent were sentenced for drug violations. As of 2007, an estimated 6,487 American lives had been lost from the direct consequences of the war on drugs (extremely conservative estimate). If overdoses and the cost of this country's paralyzing drug laws are counted the number rises to 15,000 lives lost (overdoses are mostly due to the unregulated and unpredictable quality of illegal drugs, which results in dosing mistakes).

As early as 1996 the editors of The **National Review**, traditionally one of the most highly respected forums for conservative thought in America, issued a unilateral statement condemning the war on drugs; "**National Review** has not, until now, opined formally on the subject. We do so at this point. To put off a declarative judgment would be morally and intellectually weak-kneed. .....it is our judgment that the war on drugs has failed, that it is diverting intelligent energy away from how to deal with the problem of addiction, that it is wasting our resources, and that it is encouraging civil, judicial, and penal procedures associated with police states. We all agree on movement toward legalization, even though we may differ on just how far."[36] From this it seems clear that deep concern about the war on drugs runs across liberal and conservative political lines. There is a large amount of support for decriminalization or legalization of psychoactive substances, generally *not because some form of legalization and regulation offers a perfect remedy for addiction (it does not), but because the war on drugs, as is, is so very destructive to our society and our population.* An obvious consequence of legal regulation and quality control of psychoactive substances might be that it would delimit overdose deaths due to contaminated or 'bad drugs'. And redirecting a significant portion of the money now devoted to the war on drugs to the treatment of addictions and realistic education about drugs and abuse could have a huge positive impact on the wellbeing and health of our population. It likely would result in a significant reduction in the number of addictions. In place of jobs lost in the areas of drug enforcement, the penal and corrections industry, and other associated industries, other jobs in the areas of treatment, education, and regulation of legalized drugs would be created. The criminal enterprises created by the demand for illegal drugs might dry up almost completely. Deaths directly associated with the war on drugs could be virtually eradicated. How to implement this regulated legalization and some kind of legitimate, state of the art, government backed treatment regime would need to be worked out carefully, probably by referring to and utilizing the significant body of research already completed on treatment methods and outcomes, and then perhaps by trial and error. But it would at least reduce the damage done by the present program.

So why is the war on drugs such an entrenched and seemingly immovable abomination? It is estimated that legalization of drugs could reduce the necessary size of all police agencies in the nation by one-third.[35] In 2003 that would have amounted to 12.9 billion dollars saved on local police agencies alone. Add another $9 billion in domestic and international law enforcement and the number rises to $21.9 billion. Considering prison expenses, for year 2007 the estimated total amount spent by federal and state prisons on costs associated with the drug war was $30.4 billion. Obviously, many thousands of jobs are dependent on the war on drugs, and the proposed changes threaten the security of those jobs. But it is beyond disgusting to realize that those jobs are created by legal policies which produce crime instead of reducing it, cause addiction instead of stopping it, cost thousands of lives and ruin many thousands more. The salaries for these jobs are paid for by the very people who wind up being harmed by the policies they pay to support. In plain terms, the war on drugs is an artificially manufactured industry which is paid for by all of the citizens of our nation, whom it victimizes.

At this advanced point in the history of the war on drugs, a huge amount of information and telling statistics have been accrued, with strong opposition from a majority of our most brilliant experts in the field. For governments, congressmen, police officials, rehabilitation and penal officials, and a multitude of other seemingly intelligent leaders to resist change by claiming that legalization offers no certitude or proven outcome is ludicrous. At the very least, the numbers of lives lost as a direct result of the war on drugs would certainly have to decrease if the war on drugs is removed. There is no perfect solution for addiction any more than there is a perfect solution for diabetes or many other disease syndromes. However, we can at least stop doing what we know is destructive. The incidence of illegal drug abuse and crime related to illegal drugs simply continues to increase,[37] regardless of how much money and manpower we pour into the effort to curtail supply. The war on drugs simply does not work. It is another example of our government's attempt to oversimplify problems by reducing them to the lowest common denominator, things. This criminalization of drugs *suggests* to people that there must be something very *alluring* about drugs for them to be deemed illegal. The present legal policy focuses on crime, whereas the treatment of addictions needs to focus on the disease process. Doing something illegal is generally much more alluring than doing something sick or associated with disease. Keeping drugs completely illegal actually teases our population with questions about how drug experiences must feel. It is obvious to virtually everyone that many people have used drugs and not gotten arrested. And often they have used drugs more than once. Almost every person, from teenage on up, has known or been acquainted with someone who has used illegal substances. Simply making drugs illegal has not kept their use and availability out of the public eye. But this illegality keeps the focus on crime, not the disease.

To be clear, the war on drugs helps create and perpetuate addiction in our culture by encouraging people to focus on *things*, the drugs, instead of the real problem, which is the disease of addiction. Every kind of mental problem is actually a problem with *processes*, not things. The problem exists in the *relationship* to things, not because the things merely exist. Our nation *must* end the war on drugs or it will continue to distract us from the true pathology of addiction inside our society; and it will continue to get worse. In simple terms, if we just put forth a reasonable committed effort, it would be difficult for us to create a new policy involving legalization, regulation, and intense treatment for addiction which *could* be as destructive as the war on drugs. The new program might be troubling, complex, difficult, far from perfect, but easily better than what we have now. A humane ethical and moral standard which focuses on care and effective treatment of our populace, and one which focuses on saving lives and nurturing health, would allow us to feel *right* about our nation's intentions. The artificial and arbitrary war on drugs misses the point and leaves us feeling conflicted, disgusted, and demoralized because of our government's destructive actions.

PART TWO

The Perfect Solution & The Only Way Out

"Where there is ultimate concern, God can be denied only in the name of God. One God can deny the other one."

Paul Tillich 1886-1965

9

Essential Addiction and Essential Wellness

Sam Schumacher, an Episcopal priest in the 1930s who worked with alcoholics, stated that, "Alcoholics suffer the divine restlessness from which the saints are made. It keeps them moving, striving, reaching out."[38] By now it may be obvious that the whole point of addiction is substitute satisfaction; that is, it attempts to use artificial fixes for an essential *something* that is lacking inside the person. Usually the addict either does not know (cannot conceptualize) what the lacking essence might be, or does not believe that it can actually be attained in the real world. In either case, the addict lacks accurate knowledge of the missing element and knowledge of what healthy living really is. Often the addict has never experienced real peace or happiness, and consequently is naïve and/or ignorant about its existence in the lives of healthy people. And when they hear people talk about it, they often think that the person is making up superficial stories for the sake of self-aggrandizement. Or when the addict hears someone mention peacefulness, he/she assumes that means that everything in the other person's life is working so smoothly that relaxation automatically occurs, not realizing that relaxation and peace are conscious choices in spite of how smoothly things are going. Or, for instance, the average addict does not believe that intuition, as a legitimate way of discerning reality, is viable. The addict attributes all intuition to simple coincidence, not surprising in our materialistic cause-and-effect world. When the addict sees or hears of someone else's happy love relationship, seemingly without problems or contention, the addict assumes that person must have a partner who agrees with everything their mate says or does, not realizing that good relationships need to be maintained through negotiation. The addict, in general, has little appreciation or knowledge of life as process and negotiation. In his/her mind life works mechanistically, similar to billiard balls on a pool table interacting with each other in straight-line cause-and-effect fashion. There is little appreciation for the value of emotions in the addict's life. The concept of intimacy is typically reduced mostly to sex. In the eyes of the addict, happiness can only be attained through *doing,* not *being.* The theories and research mentioned earlier, about life actually being transcendent, transpersonal, and mediated by consciousness itself, are typically foreign to the addict. The addict, even if nominally religious, believes that mysticism, transcendence, and transpersonal connection is for another life (perhaps an afterlife), but not for this one. He/she typically believes that God, spirit, higher power, or mystical presence is *out there* somewhere (perhaps heaven), but is not an indwelling presence *inside* each of us at all times, not an inherent part of humanity. And if the addict does believe in a higher power out there, he/she usually believes that they must somehow coax the higher power to come to them; that they are somehow detached from it unless it chooses to communicate with them.

This fatalistic, antiquated, hyper-materialistic view of reality is at the heart of addiction. It misconstrues reality similar to the way the inquisition misconstrued reality when it forced Galileo to recant his support for the theory that the earth moves around the sun, that the earth is not the center of the universe. Clinging to the antiquated idea that reality is only material things is not just limiting, it is disastrous. Newtonian physics is dead as an explanation for how reality-at-large works. To be clear, we must, of course, work out our existence in the everyday world of material things. But it is impossible to attain *meaningful* existence by dealing only with the material world. We must, indeed, wear the world like a loose garment, realizing that true meaningfulness can only be had in peaceful interaction with other people and with the life force, which is beneath, within, between, and beyond all things.

These words, concepts, theories, and results of research will not sound unusual to many of our citizens who have grown up in a religious environment. The idea of a transcendent reality, something which exceeds the material world, has been the essential aspect of the theology and teaching of almost all religions. Churches and religions have been the primary teachers for passing on moral and ethical lessons and encouraging constructive care and love for others in our culture since the founding of our nation. These teachings and traditions have been the basic principles which have helped guard our nation from being overwhelmed by addictive degeneration up to the present day.

The essential remedy for the problem of addiction is mystical or spiritual or transcendent experience, which results in a new metaphysical understanding of the world. However, a hidden part of the addiction process sometimes exists *in* churches and within almost all denominations and religions to some extent. Like all human institutions, churches and organized religions continually are forced to create policies designed to deal with recurring issues, and to define their standards, and to specify what their beliefs and values are. This necessarily results in rules, regulations, and policies for conducting the business and life of the church. These choices are unavoidable in the day-to-day material world. But these regulations, policies and rules have often resulted in dogma which *excludes,* rather than *includes,* other people and religions. Churches, like individuals, cannot be everything to everyone. That is not humanly possible. However, when religions and churches do not strive toward acceptance of others (err in the direction of love instead of fear), then the very *concept* of a God who is the mediator of all of reality is precluded by limitation. These acts of exclusion put human limits on the concept which by definition has no limits. *Fear* is the main contaminating ingredient which drives some churches and religions to be over-controlling and exclusive. In the same way that fear creates prejudice in general, fear creates prejudice in religion, fear which is antithetical to the very idea of love, compassion, and sharing (love your neighbor as yourself). The net result is that religion, in some cases, can result in distortion and denigration of healthy, holistic spirituality. Churches and religions sometimes *thingify* spirituality by attempting to reduce it to rules, limits, and arbitrary human rituals. In this process, the very essence of transcendence can be lost by reducing it to the mundane and superficial. To be clear, our churches and our religious traditions have definitely been the standard bearers and purveyors of all that is fine and good in America. They have saved us from ourselves over and over throughout our history. However, we must not lose sight of the fact that the regulation of spirituality in order to provide rules for religion is an extremely delicate and dangerous process. In today's world, with our society's huge motivation for thingifying, marketing, packaging, and commercializing almost everything, our religious institutions and our spiritual heritage are under a greater threat than ever from those same forces which threaten mental health. The attempt to thingify all of reality is, indeed, a direct affront to our religious and spiritual heritage.

The missing piece for the addict is *personal spiritual experience*. However, the addict's mystical reorganization of life might not fit with organized religion's traditional definitions of spiritual experience. Obviously, what is implied by this new experience is a change in the way the addict views reality and what life means. It is, of course, a new start on a new life for the addict. But it sometimes appears in a very personalized or idiosyncratic way, not necessarily religious but nevertheless spiritual.

It can be confusing, in our black and white/on or off society to understand just where addiction begins, and what qualifies a person as an addict. There are those persons who have experienced periods (sometimes long periods) of continual abuse of substances and/or behaviors who manage to moderate their behavior or quit without great difficulty. While their obsessive–compulsive actions would qualify them as addicts, they somehow, often without intervention or without obvious difficulty, reorganize their lives relatively gracefully. Perhaps they find new life meaning accidentally, or do not have any genetic predisposition for addiction. Or perhaps they simply mature over time, or have been fortunate enough to have wise supporters and loved ones, who have modeled for the addict what real happiness is without pushing the addict to change. However, the more severely addicted person usually has to hit a very low ebb in her/his life (hit bottom) before they are willing to seriously consider stopping the addictive behaviors and actually question what they believe about life. For this person, in order for recovery to occur, the new mystical experience may come in a flash of awareness (like the burning bush). Or it may come in a slower and more gradual growing awareness, which comes out of practicing living in a new way. That experiential learning which comes from practice often leads to a new kind of insight and new beliefs and attitudes. In either case, the addict will become aware that a true miracle has happened in his/her life. It most often takes the help of others who have some knowledge and/or personal experience of recovery to guide the addict through this process. The addict will no longer need the addictive substance or behavior to cope, and eventually life will become happier than they could have imagined. Perhaps the most important thing to understand is that the addict's whole life must change for recovery to continue, not just the removal of the main symptom(s), the addictive substances(s), and/or the addictive behavior(s). Recovery from pathological addiction necessitates a total life reorganization.

Essential wellness can, to some degree, be deduced from the explanation above. The ability to avoid and overcome addiction is a major part of mental health. Mental health is a relative concept, which describes an ongoing process. It ebbs and flows, increases and diminishes, and is dependent on a great number of factors. Mental health necessitates, most of all, a rich sense of life meaning, a belief in something which transcends the individual self and transcends material reality.

It takes an appreciation of the value of life, which cannot be expressed in simple rational terms. Good mental health necessitates a recognition that life is process and story, a continual unfolding revelation of reality arrived at through experience. Those who value life practice rigorous honesty for the sake of fairness, compassion, and support for all of life, not just their own. Some members of our population have been fortunate enough to have been brought up in families and circumstances which promote and teach this rich view of life. Often their beliefs and attitudes are strong due to a lifetime of practice. They provide a resilient backbone of strength and care for the society as a whole. However, some of these lack insight and compassion for other members of our society who have not grown up in the same fortunate circumstances. Some may not be able to appreciate the huge stress, if not trauma, of discovering that the beliefs of a lifetime are incorrect. They may not be able to appreciate having to completely reorganize how one lives and what one believes in order to recover from problems inherited from out-of-balance parents or a chaotic, abusive upbringing. Those of our population without sufficient socialization (or incorrect socialization) are the most at risk for addiction, but none of us are immune.

Robust mental health necessitates some understanding and an appreciation of emotion as a necessary element of life. Emotions are what make each of us unique and also what make us similar to one another. Intimacy is a must for happiness, and it can happen easily or with difficulty, depending on the person's comfort with his/her own emotions. Intimacy is based on the ability to share emotion openly and transparently. It is so important precisely because it is how we share our true humanity, our real lives with each other. Intimacy is the glue which holds people together, because it provides the forum for us to say and hear how it feels to be alive. Without intimacy, which may be attained in many ways, loneliness would ultimately overwhelm us. Real intimacy (not pseudo-intimacy) also necessitates rigorous honesty. Pseudo-intimacy is the 'drug' of codependency, and is present in most other addictions as well. Pseudo-intimacy acts intimately in the same way an actor plays a role, on an as-if basis. It is not real.

Essential mental health necessitates the recognition that healthy relationships are built on negotiation. Good relationships do not necessarily come from people being very similar to each other, although some common interests are necessary. Good relationships come from people being willing to share their emotions honestly, and negotiating agreements with each other for the satisfaction of individual and mutual needs and wishes. Good boundaries make for good relationships of all kinds. The responsibility of partners in any kind of relationship is to reveal their own needs and wishes to the other. It is not the responsibility of partners in relationship to try to discover or discern or learn the wishes of the other by having to question or investigate or uncover information which is not forthcoming. Each of us has the responsibility to inform others of what we need and want. It is not the responsibility of the other person to pry it out of us. Again, rigorous honesty and the courage to be real is the issue.

Essential mental health necessitates the ability to be still and to practice peace. People who are mentally healthy are human beings, not just human doings. The inability to turn off the internal dialogue and be still is perhaps the most pervasive symptom of addiction in our culture. Americans are said to work harder as a nation than virtually anyone else in the world. What we do not do well is relax. A majority of the people in our society do not know how to be still, at least not inside, not in the mind. Many people do not know how to be alone and at peace within, because our society is one that thrives on competition. It emphasizes competition relentlessly. Consequently, a person must always be moving, or at least be planning to move. We are taught to believe that we must stay constantly prepared and ready. Life is seen as a contest, with only winners and losers. Think of how much pressure there is for winning or scoring high, even when playing games or sports where the goal is supposed to be *fun*. Healthy competition is, of course, a necessity and can be pleasurable, but our culture fosters competition so unrelentingly that it has become an obsession. The result of this almost exclusive kind of focus, living for competition, is that we continually practice being adversaries. We do not learn relaxation and cooperative relationship; we learn work, hyper-vigilance, and fear. Ultimately, as a society, we do not learn peace, we learn war. The essentially mentally healthy person knows and practices relaxation and peace, plays well and celebrates life, has a deep understanding of life as being, not just doing, has a sense of life as much larger than just her/his self and feels connected intimately to the life force. The healthy person feels ultimately free to express his/her uniqueness and ultimately connected and similar to all of humanity at the same time. This kind of life requires not only some intellectual understanding of a holistic frame for reality, but also some experiential knowledge. This has to happen by putting academic knowledge ('head' knowledge) into action ('experiential' knowledge). What we have actually experienced is what we really believe. The mentally healthy person is at peace with him/her self, because he/she is not hiding from anyone, including his/her self. This person sees life as an exploration, and is in love with all of life, from the largest overarching aspects (God or the life force) to the individual (self and other) coping with life on life's terms day by day.

10

Attention and Peacefulness

Learning to stop, to be still, and to quieten the frenetic mind is perhaps the most difficult task necessary to accomplish peace. To learn to *be*, not just to *do*, is essential for life reorganization, so that recovery from addiction can occur. Learning to be peaceful, in and with ourselves, is the essential ingredient of robust mental health. The only way we can experience the *being* side of life is to learn to stop living exclusively in the material world, the *doing* world. Most of us have had a whole lifetime of living in the material world, continually moving, working, seeking, and striving to attain security and predictability for ourselves and our families. Even our play is most often dominated by doing instead of being. Most individuals and our society as a whole have an addictive habit of unrest. This robs from us the ability to experience the world spiritually. It robs us of the ability to discover our true selves. It robs us of the ability to sense and share our emotions; intimacy is limited. It robs us of the ability to be optimally creative, because creativity, in general, is conceptualizing outside of the boundaries of the average everyday world. It robs us of relaxation, because we cannot stop and be still. It keeps us addicted to the past, because we do not know how to stop and shift into new modes of being and thinking. It robs us of the knowledge of peace, so that we continue to practice adversarial thinking, focusing on the other instead of the self.

Many in our society have experienced peace only rarely or accidentally and consequently are not really familiar with peace in their personal lives. Some of us actually fear peace, because it appears to imply a state of nothingness. For forty years as a practicing psychologist, I have been asking clients what they believe would happen if they actually stopped thinking by turning off the internal dialogue, not using words or ideas to analyze experiences, but simply practiced *being*. A large number of them have reported that they believe they would go completely out of control (lose their minds). A few have even reported that they believe they would die. This inherent fear of having to go without words for even a short while demonstrates that a significant number of our population are slaves to their inner voices. Self talk is, of course, necessary. It is the machinery necessary for thinking, calculating, planning, judging, discerning and manipulating material reality. However, words are manmade symbols, at least once removed from the actual things and issues of the world. Words provide an arbitrary map of the sensate world, but are not capable of capturing *ultimate* or *whole* reality. We must utilize a different technique to approach holistic reality.

There is a solution to this problem. It has to do with learning to focus attention. Virtually all of the world's great spiritual traditions teach some sort of focus of attention through the use of meditation exercises. There are many different forms of meditation, and they may seem very different from one another at first glance. However, they all have the same ultimate purpose; they teach control of attention.[39], [40], [41], [42], [43] That ability to focus attention provides the tool necessary to turn off the internal dialogue and be quiet. The control of attention has at least two essential elements: the ability to hold attention in one place and the ability to shift attention at will. These two elements are the basic psychological functions necessary to submit to the things we cannot change (live life on life's terms), and to exercise the will to change the things we can (exchange bad habits for good ones). No other psychological ability is so necessary in order to achieve true balance in life. Meditation is the primary tool to learn this control. In general, meditation exercises instruct the meditator to focus *all* of the attention on some singular object, sound, word, or very simple concept. This object of attention can be thought of as a kind of perceptual *singularity.* It should be something that is so fundamental that it cannot be further analyzed into pieces (such as a dot on a blank wall).

Meditation is both a goal in and of itself and also a tool to help us learn to control attention. Meditation, in the ideal sense, is pure sensation without words or ideas to filter the experience. Meditation is a *goal* in that it opens us to the experience of oneness with all of reality without any object or boundary in the way to distract us. This is the antithesis of everyday reality. This may seem contradictory at first glance, because most forms of meditation use some material object or point to focus on (the singularity). However, it operates on the principle that, if *all* of the attention is focused on the singularity, no attention will be left over to distract us with other thoughts or objects of attention. The singularity must be so simple and psychologically basic that it cannot be reduced intellectually to smaller pieces or elements. Items such as a dot on the wall, a pure tone, a very basic sensation such as the feeling in the end of the finger, or a simple repetitive action such as running or walking at a steady pace are examples of things which can be used for meditation (more on this later). Meditation is a *tool* in that it teaches us to focus attention where we choose, and to not be distracted or seduced by those things which we cannot control. The ultimate goal is to *live life as a meditation*; that is, to live every moment (or at least most moments) in conscious awareness that we must move *with* the flow of the river of life, not against it. This necessitates raised consciousness and willful choice. Meditation helps us learn the new habits necessary to carry this out.

The basic idea of meditation to achieve peacefulness is actually very simple. It has to do with the very definition of the word *meditation*. Meditation is often confused with prayer. Prayer may be conceptualized as *talking* to God or the higher power, while meditation may be conceptualized as *listening*, listening not just with the ears, but with all the senses, the mind, the body, and the heart all at once. In order to achieve this whole awareness it is necessary to *turn off* the internal dialogue, to stop talking to one's self. This can be accomplished by focusing *all* of the attention on some singular thing, so that there is no attention left over to distract us into self talk. The point is to stay absolutely in the present moment, in the eternal *now.*

What we use as a focus for our attention in meditation is not so important as long as we follow a few simple guidelines. The focus of attention can involve virtually any of the human sense modalities and even some limited mental modalities. The image, word(s), symbol, sound, mantra, feeling, or repetitive action used as the singularity for focusing attention should be simple or profound (as opposed to complex or intricate). It should be constructive and/or peaceful in quality (as opposed to destructive, fearful, or agitating). Some examples of the kinds of things used for meditation include counting breaths (like counting sheep, but start over after you count to four or five); focusing on a body part or feeling (as in some forms of yoga); the use of a mantra (or sound) which is repeated over and over in the mind; the repetition of a very short prayer (shorter is better, even just one word); focusing on a *koan* or riddle (simple, such as the color of the wind, or the sound of one hand clapping); focusing on an icon or some simple visual artifact: focusing on the image of some meaningful symbol (such as the image of a flame); using some repetitive action such as running or swimming (but the mind must be held on the action, or attention will begin to wander). There is also at least one method of meditation which takes the totally opposite approach: it teaches the meditator to notice everything that comes through the mind, but to let it pass immediately, to not cling on to things (this meditation is perhaps more difficult for beginners). From the above suggestions, it should be obvious that there are many traditional forms of meditation, and still others may be created on an individual basis. The goal of the practice is to hold attention in one place and not be distracted, and to shift attention only when the meditator chooses to do so.

The ultimate goal, of course, is not simply to learn to do meditation exercises, but to learn through the practice to reach a natural harmony with the world. This harmony produces a self confidence (trust in ultimate reality) so that we cannot be deluded or seduced into addiction to the artificial things and ideas which surround us. The real life experience of an uncluttered mind knows the path to peace and constructive living innately. It does not cling to things or people fearfully; it lives and lets live. Training in meditation is training for a more natural lifestyle.

Routine practice of at least a few minutes each day is necessary in the beginning. Fifteen to thirty minutes most days is enough for learning to develop. However, some spiritual traditions recommend much more rigorous practice for longer periods each day. Practicing some form of relaxation may be useful before each meditation session. . Relaxation can remove the distractions of tense muscles and *noise* from the body. Some meditators may prefer to adhere to the rules for meditation of a specific spiritual tradition, while others may view their practice as an independent personal adventure into peacefulness and harmony. It may be helpful for the individual to try a few different techniques in order to find one which fits her/him best. However, training in meditation is not easy, and the meditator should expect progress to be slow at first, and never perfect even with advanced training. Most students can only maintain their focus of attention for a few minutes at a time in the beginning. It is necessary to be gentle with one's self; attention wanders off the focus point even for advanced meditators. Simply return the attention to the focus point and proceed. Never criticize yourself for wandering off focus. Don't fall into the trap of trying to *control* your meditative progress. Progress in meditation cannot be forced. We must open ourselves to it and gently *allow* our progress to grow. There is a natural innate awareness or intuition which urges us on to this goal. Ultimately we will thrive if we submit to it.

It is one of the true paradoxes of life that, that which we need the most for the survival of our society and our nation also turns out to be the most rewarding tool for living we can attain personally. The experiential knowledge of life which comes from the practice of meditation provides *subjective* awareness of life firsthand, without the filter of *objective* conceptualizations and intellectualizations in the way. This venture into our own primal reality inevitably unveils an exquisite care for all of life, energetic and childlike. It reveals the inherent wisdom of peace accrued through the experience of human beings throughout all the ages of time which precede us. This personal awareness is necessary to recover from the addictive tentacles of our society. It provides the very habits, attitudes, and true knowledge of life necessary to help thwart corruption and dishonesty in the society at large.

11

Changing Thinking, Habits, and Beliefs

Considering the ways in which addiction works (and the corruption which creates it), what mental health and mental illness actually are, the new aspects of reality revealed by science (similar to spiritual traditions), the old revealed truths of the great spiritual traditions (similar to new science), the benefits of meditation, the value of peacefulness, and the many implications of this information, what kind of holistic picture of life does this produce? This was George's question; 'how can I live as one person with my feet in two different worlds?' We might paraphrase, how can a person maintain sanity while trying to live in two different realities at the same time? There are several different answers to this question. The most basic answer might be that the overarching ultimate reality proposed by the spiritual traditions and by science is *primary*. Everyday reality is *secondary* and only an illusory reflection of the primary. Science has demonstrated that everyday reality is very pliable, transient, and malleable. Material reality, and the future which seems to unfold before us, are actually quite amenable to our wishes and personal desires. That is, everyday material reality is not nearly so hard and deterministic as it seems. This answer suggests that humans should probably pay the most attention to primary reality. Meditation has shown us that being still, shutting down our self talk, and listening with all our senses will generally provide the most direct experience of primary reality. That is, when we stop trying to *do* reality and try instead to *be* reality. The goal is to make as much of life as possible a meditation, to *be here now* as much as possible, whatever we are doing. Addiction is dependent on the inner self-talk to keep the victim enslaved. But, for the person who has learned meditation and can turn off the inner dialogue more of the time, the slave driver (self-talk) is circumvented and loses the power to enslave the would-be addict. When we can turn off the inner dialogue, we can experience reality directly. Every flower then offers the opportunity for realization of the ultimate, because we have the power to merge with it in appreciation of the life force. Meditation teaches us to drop the boundaries between our selves and the rest of reality. Boundaries are only maintained by *objectifying* the world; they are the manmade product of language and analytic thinking. This explanation is at least as old as the story from the Bible about Adam and Eve and the tree of knowledge. A modern day analogue of this story is that humans created all of the words in the world and laid them on top of the already-existing reality like a map. But humans became confused and began to treat the map as if it were the actual reality (confuse the map for the territory). Humans began to expend all of their energy and time focusing on the map, forgetting that reality was actually something different, which could be codified in different ways with different maps (other languages). At this point humans became addicted because they had reduced life to the study of the arbitrary pieces of the map and ignored the true seamless whole of reality; they were out of touch with reality. The point is not that all humans are addicts by virtue of our using language; but that the seeds of addiction are implicit in the use of manmade schemes to codify, classify, organize, and index the increments of perception. We humans tend to forget that words are at least once removed from the actual realities. In many cases the definitions of words are very arbitrary. That is the reason why different languages are sometimes not easily translated one to another. Meditation is the tool to relearn contact with true reality, because it teaches us to turn off the talk. Living meditatively is never forgetting that the map is not the real territory.

Another answer is that primary reality has to do with *being,* while secondary reality has to do with *doing.* Primary reality is not time bound according to science and the church. Primary reality is eternal or steady-state. Secondary reality can only exist in a goal oriented, sequential, time dependent way. We humans apparently need the illusion of time and space in order to provide the illusion of separateness, the autonomy of things and entities, and our ability to manipulate the world. While we humans do seem to have the capacity to initiate changes in our world, the basic underlying question is whether and when we as individuals actually *cause* changes to occur. Or is it possible that our control is sometimes an illusion; that, at least occasionally, we simply anticipate change, participate in it, and then own responsibility for the change, even though we did not personally cause it to happen? A number of experiments in physics demonstrate that the elements of reality, even though separated by vast distances, are still connected to each other in intimate, integral ways that transcend the boundaries of time and space. For instance, there is a phenomenon in physics called *quantum entanglement.*[42] It shows that if a subatomic particle, a proton for instance, is split into two sub-particles which move away from each other, each of the sub-particles will have a movement called *spin.* The spin of one sub-particle will be opposite and complementary to the other sub-particle. However, if the spin of one of the sub-particles is arbitrarily reversed, the spin of the other will also reverse instantaneously, faster than the speed of light. This has been demonstrated to occur even if the sub-particles are miles apart when the reversal occurs. The main point to gather here is that the change occurs *instantaneously.* The change in one of the sub-particles cannot be said to *cause* the change in the other; they both change at *exactly* the same time. They are connected as if they are still one particle. Our autonomy as individuals, or to what degree we actually are autonomous, is called into question by this research. This research seems to be a demonstration that primary reality ultimately prevails, that in the end, when all is said and done, we are really one and the same being. The inescapable facts of life demonstrated by this commonly accepted research (the experiments have been repeated many times) place further emphasis on the necessity for humans to be adept at living in primary reality as well as the secondary everyday world.

Another aspect to consider in answer to George's question is the value of peace in and of itself. First of all, does the practice of meditation and being quiet actually get us peace? Does focusing on the here and now and merging with the one whole reality automatically result in learning to be more peaceful? This question has an answer with two sides. One side is the subjective personal experience of peacefulness, which is in fact a direct consequence of being still in the mind, body, and spirit all at the same time. Meditation does result directly in learning *personal* peace. But, does personal peace automatically translate into *interpersonal* peace, and then international peace? In other words, does learning to be peaceful as an individual automatically indicate or imply that individuals will be peaceful with others? Most individuals report that the experience of personal tranquility which comes from meditation does result in appreciation and love for the life force in general. As a practicing psychologist teaching meditation I have seen this happen to many hundreds of individuals. Therefore, in my experience, there appears to be a very direct connection between the practice of meditation and peacefulness with self and others. However, in the history of psychology, humans were once thought to be instinctively destructive and warlike. Sigmund Freud, in 1920, proposed the theory of the death wish or death drive, *thanatos* (not Freud's word, but added by one of his students), stating that humans have an instinctive drive toward destruction and death (the opposite of peacefulness and constructiveness).[45] Freud pointed to the seemingly perpetual state of wars between various nations, and he justified his theory by pointing out the territorial disputes between lower animals. The study of animal behavior, ethology, was in its infancy at the time of Freud, and like the beginnings of virtually all sciences, the first phenomena to come up for study are the most obvious and sensational. In the case of animal behavior, some of the most extraordinary behaviors are the territorial disputes, particularly between large mammals, which are occasionally injurious or even deadly to the participants. Freud used this as evolutionary evidence to support his theory of *thanatos,* noting that humans also are mammals, and therefore we must have inherited the instinct for violence in our genes. However, we now know that the percentage of injurious territorial disputes among animals is actually very low, simply because we have been able to accrue much more observation and research with various animal species. In 1986, a group of twenty distinguished scientists from around the world, including psychologists, biologists, geneticists, sociologists, anthropologists, ethologists, psychiatrists, and others met in Seville, Spain and issued the Seville Statement on Violence. The purpose was to proclaim that it is *incorrect* scientifically to conclude that humans are preprogrammed biologically, genetically, or psychologically to be violent.[46] They concluded that war is a product of mind, and peace can be created by the mind just as easily. Freud's conclusions concerning violence were totally incorrect.

Further evidence for the conceptualization of reality in a primary and secondary configuration comes from the study of neuropsychology and brain function. British neuroscientist Iain McGilchrist has written extensively on the differing functions of the two hemispheres of the brain.[47] He has drawn together insights from a multitude of different research projects, and he details the development of knowledge about split-brain function through history. His conclusions are surprisingly (or not) similar to the picture I have tried to paint here. The right side of the brain sees the world in holistic terms, as an undivided and primary (or primal) reality. It tends to be mediated by intuitions, emotions, creative impressions, and is not necessarily rational in its functions. It keeps close contact with primary reality, which is timeless, and transcends space and individuality. It is *subjective* in its existence, maintaining the domain of *being.* The left hemisphere gradually evolved to cope with the material world in more precise, predictable ways. It is mediated by language and mathematics, logical processes which provide the predictability and security which come from planning and calculating. It is *objective* in its approach to reality, standing outside and looking back at the self and reality in general as objects. It is the thing maker, which divides reality into pieces, and creates the necessity for time, space, and individual autonomy. The left brain arose in service to the right. It is secondary, both in terms of the picture it paints of reality and in terms of evolution (it came second). However, as McGilchrist points out, over time the left brain has seized so much attention that the right hemisphere is at risk of being overpowered. We are now left with a worldview that is mechanistic, materialistic, and thing oriented, qualities which are out of touch with happiness, intimacy, creativity, and play, the qualities which really make us human.

This leaves us with the realization, based on incontrovertible facts, that we have not only the opportunity for increasing and deepening our health at all levels through the practice of personal peace. We also have a real option for the attainment of true happiness and the development of balanced, caring, and constructive relationships with others.

12

New Life Experience

So, what does it really mean to live moment-to-moment and day-to-day wearing the world like a loose garment? What does the experience feel like? What are some of the steps to this dance, and what might be some of the points of interest along the way? What I have offered so far is essentially two different ways of doing and being which are polar opposites: stillness or action, doing or being, objective and subjective, future orientation or present orientation, thinking or feeling, and other similar polarities. Is there anything in between these two extremes? We need to be able to make conscious choices about when to move and when to be still. Part of the solution lies in the ability to *be here now*, to be present and basically undistracted no matter what we do. Addiction and chaotic living are mostly the result of a cluttered mind and unceasing, chattering self-talk. Unbridled self-talk becomes a slave driver constantly trying to juggle ideas, goals, memories, and other aspects of mind as if it were totally responsible for making life happen all by itself. It clings to ideas, memories and concepts as if they surly would be lost if the person stops talking and thinking about them. Many thoughts are typically repeated over and over in the self-talk, often using exactly the same words. Unbridled self-talk, without the person realizing what is happening, typically turns into a number of obsessive compulsive repetitions of the same thoughts over and over. Sometimes the thoughts are small sentences or phrases, while other times they are large or complex conceptualizations, but they are repeated so often that they essentially fill up the mental experience of the person. However, in spite of the clinging, obsessive thinking of the addicted mind, often this mind can be easily distracted or pulled off task by extraneous unimportant thoughts or other phenomena. Both of these features of thinking are usually driven by some level of anxiety or unrest. The addicted mind is not happy with the *status quo*.

Consequently it clings onto things to try to avoid loss, but it also is somewhat hyper-vigilant in order to not miss opportunities for resolving the unrest. This can result in distraction. The underlying unrest is the key to understanding this noisy, clinging, goal oriented, chatter. The restless mind attempts to be a *human doing.* However, the restlessness cannot be resolved with mere thinking and doing.

There are at least two answers to this seeming contradiction between doing and being. Living in both worlds is inevitable, but we must learn to prioritize the steps of the journey differently than our society teaches. The real goal is peace. The peaceful (opposite of restless) mind does not need the clinging, which characterizes the addicted mind. Nor does it need to be hyper-vigilant, because it is not anxious. The ability to be peaceful implies a self-confidence in the sense that the person is confident in his/her ability to *turn on* peace, to be still and to hold the attention where he/she chooses. There is knowledge involved, and knowledge necessitates experience. The practice of meditation provides the experience and the learning necessary to stop the inner dialogue. The intellectual understanding of how reality really works, discussed earlier in previous chapters, the huge fund of scientific knowledge from physics as well as all of the life sciences, provides another kind of knowledge. The main theme of all of the great spiritual traditions (one God, or one Reality) provides yet another piece of knowledge to under-gird the goal of letting go, practicing stillness, and living peace. In reality, all is one. We are not actually separate from one another. There is only one *Being,* one *God*, one reality. I am *It*; you are *It* too; and the life force is *It.* Separateness is an illusion; the secondary reality is responsible for the creation of autonomous entities. When words and language are allowed to dominate consciousness, the result is separateness of things, people and concepts. The essence of addiction and related problems of mental illness is the belief that reality is limited to the secondary *thing* world. The craving of addiction is a misguided craving for the *experience* of something that is missing from the awareness of the addict. When humans cannot let go of language (self-talk), they are by definition *addicted* to the world of separate things. The craving is actually the longing for wholeness, for joining with the *One*, for submitting to peaceful union with the *Life Force*, for completion. For humans, nothing else but this joining with the whole can fulfill that longing.

The second part of the solution calls for a new way (actually old) to talk and conceptualize, one which is not constricted by logic or by what we typically call *reason*. The holistic breadth of theology and the new science cover territory which cannot be grasped with the standard everyday language of the manifest world. Obviously, the problem with unceasing self-talk occurs because the language is primarily content-oriented, constantly reducing reality to things. Reducing the world to things attempts to freeze-frame reality, reducing it to a series of rigid succinct snap shots. As pointed out earlier, every facet of reality is involved in the life process. For instance, it has been discovered that empty space everywhere actually contains lots of energy; the cosmos is essentially a continuous lattice of energy with no gaps. Every single thing is moving, changing, evolving, living, dying, and being reborn always. We at least need words and concepts which are more process-oriented, which can allude to the livingness which is life. The scientific explanations of primary reality go beyond the limits of reason, and they break the rules of logic and everyday reasoning. The spiritual and religious traditions intuitively recognized the problem from the start and bypassed rational thinking, relying on *revealed* truths instead. Finally, at present, humanity has arrived at the point where all of science and religion are essentially in agreement that ultimate, whole reality cannot be captured accurately with mere words. We need some ways to share our common experiences of it, to try to describe the *aliveness* of life experiences, and what it feels like to live in awareness of its presence. This new kind of communication, while still dependent on the words of common languages must focus on some uncommon (in our culture) aspects of reality and experience. The primary emphasis must be on subjective experience, because we have shown that ultimate reality exists outside the realm of objective descriptions; it supersedes objective descriptions. The new communication must somehow attempt to convey *personal experience.* The life force drives us toward intimacy, because intimacy is the sharing of personal experience. Personal experience is the only way we can really appreciate and communicate awareness of the *One* reality. From this perspective, life really must be lived as art. Artistic expression is dependent on very few rules, and it offers the possibility for optimum communication of subjective experience. I am not necessarily referring to the fine arts, although they certainly are prime examples of self-expression. Rather, I am suggesting that thinking, expressing, relating to others and to the world in general must go beyond the literal thingified world to include *feelings, emotions, joy, pain, love,* and those expressions which convey *life.* Humans are instinctively driven toward intimacy, toward sharing. Humans are apparently some of the most gregarious creatures on earth. We press together in cities which have larger populations than the largest anthills or the largest termite mounds. We have an instinctive need to be close, to share, and to cooperate with our own kind. We are extremely social animals. This drive is not learned, it is apparently based on pure instinct. It is in the genes. It implies directly that we are seeking to *join.* We apparently recognize instinctively that we are not truly autonomous. We are constantly attempting to act in regard to the whole, and for the benefit of the whole. Life as we know it only makes sense if it is life in relationship to others. We can deduce, therefore, that this press toward wholeness is even in our biology, not only our psychology and sociology. Practicing peace, stillness, cooperation, and love is the highest expression of this instinctive drive toward intimacy.

To live life as art is, from one perspective, to live life as story, narrative, parable, myth, and metaphor. Remembering that the essential self is eternal, not bound by time or space, not separate from the *One*, and that secondary reality is illusory, leaves us free to distance ourselves from the problems, difficulties, and delusions which have caused suffering from clinging to them. To paraphrase a Buddhist saying, 'pain is inevitable, suffering is optional'. Psychologically, because our culture teaches us to think of ourselves as autonomous beings, we tend to *own* our individual problems and pain as part of our personal autonomous identities. We have learned to objectify ourselves as things, and we think of life as what happens to that thing or to this thing as if we were talking about a machine. This causes each of us in our society to attribute his/her identity to his/her history. 'Why me?' becomes the mantra. From this point of view, each individual is bound by the past in a kind of addiction to personal history. The problem is not that we have awareness and memories of our personal history, but that we *cling* to the history as if it were the most significant defining feature of our lives. However, history is destiny only if we volunteer for it. Learning to guide and focus attention allows us to drop the burdens of the past, to stop playing the role of victim and to move into the future. Thinking of life as story is a very useful tool to separate our selves from the burdens and pain of the past. Conceptualizing life as story or narrative allows us to rewrite some things, or at least to author a new sort of story for the future. We are created by life and we are co-creators of life by virtue of the choices we make. Both science and religion tell us that conscious choice is a major element in shaping the future to suit our desires. For religion, prayer is the operational mechanism to influence the future. Science agrees when it talks about the conscious choices of the experimenter influencing the outcomes of experiments. Also, the parapsychology research on intercessory prayer having significant positive outcomes offers consensual validation for the tradition of prayer for others. Theoretically, prayer is not necessarily succinct words, but starts as a desire or wish; it is willfulness. The thing to take from this explanation is not that the future is totally shaped by our wants and wishes, but that our wants and wishes do have some significant power for influencing the future. It appears that our conscious willfulness is most powerful when it is used for *constructive* actions, actions which benefit as many people as possible, or which result in some significant benefit for an individual, but not at the expense of someone else. This argument follows (and research proves it) from the idea that we are not actually separate from one another, but exist as one in the whole.

The great psychologist Carl Jung, mentioned earlier, in some ways anticipated the need for a method to describe and communicate about life which is broader and more comprehensive than our limited cause-and-effect content oriented language. He apparently understood the usefulness of viewing life as story, myth, narrative, allegory, and metaphor. He saw that these ways of describing life are not bound by the hard rules of logic, which lock us into the thing world and keep us addicted to history. In his research and practice he focused on certain aspects of human existence which he called *archetypes.*[48] Archetypes are the most basic, most fundamental, primal conceptualizations of reality for humans. Some are as simple as a perfect circle or a perfect cross. Others characterize slightly more complex pieces of knowledge such as mother, father, earth, sea, and sky. Still others characterize basic human instincts and behaviors such as the concept of the hero, the usefulness of tools, or protection of children. There are probably hundreds or perhaps thousands of archetypes, and they provide the under-girding base, the basic roots, for the development of languages. Archetypes provide the elements which are common to all languages. Essentially, all well developed human languages contain all of the archetypal elements. Archetypes are a sort of psychological genetics. No healthy human needs to learn the archetypes; all humans are born with the knowledge of these basic ways to conceptualize life. The most important point to grasp is that the archetypes are some of the essential *instinctual* pieces of knowledge. They are wired into humans in the mechanisms of the brain. For this reason, the archetypes are *pre*logical in origin. They evolved *before* humans created formal logic and languages. Yet they provide enough elementary factual knowledge for a human to survive without learning a formal language. Jung's system of psychology, called *analytical psychology*, analyzes dreams, daydreams, reveries, fantasies, and the person's reflections on everyday experiences to find references to the underlying archetypal material. This kind of analysis obviously can be very broad in its scope and rich in its content, because it deals with reality from virtually every perceptual perspective, not just those confined to logic and reason. A good example of the archetypes, as they appear in common everyday life, is the fact that virtually every one of the common fairy tales (first recorded on paper as "Grim's Fairy Tales", but passed on verbally from generation to generation throughout history) appears in some basically similar form in virtually every human culture on earth. Further, all stories, novels, movies, and even common conversations are all based in the common archetypes which characterize humanity. The common essence in all of these is the *experience* of living. Interestingly, the *prime* archetype is God, the One, the First Concept; and the persistent urge of humans to communicate their experience to one another is in service of the instinctive drive toward unity. Our narratives describe the highest and finest actions, such as the hero's journey, which characterizes the best, most constructive things humans can do in service of other humans, for love of humankind (the whole). The anti-hero or villain characterizes the most destructive, divisive, evil, and anti-life actions we all fear and hate, because of the potential for harm to the life force. All basically decent humans are in love with life itself. Our stories and narratives are celebrations of this most profound fact of life.[49]

The summary and conclusion of all this information leads to a new kind of natural philosophy, which includes not only the material facts of nature, but the huge holistic processes and esoteric insights derived from the new science. The life force expresses itself not only in hard material reality but in the contiguous relationships between all living things and the strange processes described by physicists and cosmologists. The overwhelming conclusion is that all of life and all of reality are of one fabric. From the holistic perspective, all of life and reality is one being, unchanging, eternal, beyond the limits of time, space, and individual identity. From the materialistic and embodied perspective, all of life is connected in a web of symbiotic processes among individual persons and other living creatures and things. The whole universe is alive. These conclusions are at least as esoteric as most theologies, and seem farther afield than some science fiction novels. Nevertheless, there is a beautiful symmetry to this understanding of life. There is a tradition in science of believing that good theories and good science should offer symmetry and beauty; that there should be no contradictions. There is pleasure in the sense that *this feels right.* In other words, the basic *intuitive* insight of religion (revealed truth), which goes back to the beginning of history, now has consensual validation from the rigorous *intellectual*, mathematical and analytical machinations of science. It offers at least a basic agreement with religion in the concept of one Supreme Being. It does not, of course, agree with any specific belief or dogma of any one church or theology, nor do many of the religions agree with each other. Nevertheless, it is an astounding time in history, because for the first time in history science is in essential agreement with the church. This should offer strong evidence for church-goers, agnostics, and hard-nosed scientists alike.

For the treatment of the addictions, which are embedded so deeply in our culture, the new science offers a new tool for treatment which can be used to cut through the denial and resistance to change. The traditional fatalistic attitudes and beliefs of the addict, whether she/he pays lip service to a belief in some higher power, can resist the revealed truths offered by the church because the addict most often discounts theology as lacking proof. However, because science also now offers proof of the unity, integrity, and aliveness of the universe, and for the One-Being theory, the addict is left almost totally without any opportunity for rationalizing or intellectualizing his/her resistance to change. The dilemma for the addict is lack of power; and submitting to the fact that that he/she has no power to control addiction without help is the first step necessary to begin recovery. Acknowledging that there is some power greater than her/him self is the necessary step to open the addict to spiritual/mystical experience. The new science provides a huge new motivation to accept this view of life.

As for mental health in general, if all of the features of addiction were removed, the number of problems of life which can legitimately be qualified as mental illness would be very greatly reduced. The delusions and dishonesty associated with addiction account for an overwhelming proportion of the mental pathology in our society. The fact that our government, the pharmaceutical industry, and the medical establishment help create, feed, and perpetuate the delusions and dishonesty in our society is an outright atrocity. Those institutions which should be the cornerstones of our nation are very flawed and damaged. As with the remedy for the individual addict, the first step must be to admit to the problem and to acknowledge that we are powerless to change this societal problem with mere words. We can only change it when we as individuals choose to look beyond our individual selves to a higher power and live *genuine* lives. Truth is the only thing that will change it. We certainly do need to fight these atrocities with words, but we must *walk our talk*. It must begin with personal honesty, genuine care for our fellows, and the practice of peace.

Lives lived for the sake of competition are caught in the societal delusion that acquisition and personal status will create happiness. Those things will *not* create happiness; they will only create the need for more acquisition. To the contrary, the practice of peace is the answer, which includes and produces all of the positive remedies and aspirations for life mentioned in this book. Emulating peace is the most powerful thing in the world. Being peace is everything!

Chapter Notes and Bibliography

Chapter 1   The National Addiction: An Overview

1. George Soros *The Soros Lectures at the Central European University* (New York: Publicaffairs, 2010), 84. The writings of George Soros are a major source of information concerning the growing dishonesty in big business, politics, and the general population in the U.S.

2. _____ page 59.

3. Anne Wilson Schaef *When Society Becomes an Addict* (San Francisco: Harper & Row, Publishers, 1987). Schaef offered the first popular explanation of how addictive systems are always in play wherever there are addicts.

4. George Soros, *The Soros Lectures at the Central European University* (New York: Publicaffairs, 2010), 54

5. American Psychiatric Association *Diagnostic and Statistical Manual IV-TR* (American Psychiatric Assoc., 2000).

6. George Soros *The Soros Lectures at the Central European University* (New York: Publicaffairs, 2010), 56.

7. Donella Meadows Archive, "Why Should We Be Glad When the GNP Goes Up?" Sustainability Institute, 3 Linden Road, Hartland, VT 05048.

Chapter 2   What is Mental Health?

8. World Health Organization (2005), Promoting Mental Health: Concepts, Emerging Evidence, Practice: A Report of The World Health Organization. Geneva.

9. Personal communication.

10. Daniel J. Carlat *Unhinged, the trouble with psychiatry-A doctor's revelations about a profession in crisis.* (New York: Simon and Schuster, 2010), 7. This book is a goldmine of insight into the questionable practices of psychiatry, the drug industry, politicians, and dubious marketing practices.

11._____pages 11, 85, 119, 149.

Chapter 3   What is addiction?

12. Kevin McCauley *Pleasure Unwoven: An Explanation of the Brain Disease of Addiction* (Institute for Addiction Study, 2010), DVD. This video offers a thorough explanation of the pleasure pathways triggered by addictions.

13. John Bradshaw *Healing The Shame That Binds You* (Deerfield Beach Fla.:Health Communications Inc., 1988). This book is an excellent treatment of how shame relates to addiction.

Chapter 4   Medical versus psychological

14. Eds., John C. Norcross, Gary R. Vandenbos, and Donald K. Freedheim *The History of Psychotherapy, Continuity and Change, second edition* (Washington D.C.: American Psychological Association, 2012).

15. Daniel J. Carlat *Unhinged: The trouble With Psychiatry-A Doctor's Revelations about a Profession in Crisis* (New York: Simon and Schuster, 2010), 7. Very interesting read, but troubling.

Chapter 5   Brain versus mind

16. Gary Hatfield "Rene Descartes" in *The Stanford Encyclopedia of Philosophy* (Stanford: Center for the Study of

Language and Information, 2012). This is an open access internet resource for the study of philosophy.

17. Henry P. Stapp *Mindful Universe: Ouantum Mechanics and the Participating Observer* (New York: Springer, 2007). This book offers one of the most concise and understandable explanations of the weird quantum world.

18. Leonard Susskind *The Black Hole War: My Battle With Stephen Hawking to Make the World Safe for Quantum Mechanics* (New York: Little, Brown, and Co., 2008). Provides a state-of-the-art explanation of cosmology, modern physics, and a mind-bending picture of ultimate reality.

19. Dean Radin *The Conscious Universe* (New York: Harper Collins, 1997). Irrefutable proof about how pliable and mercurial reality actually is.

20. American Society for Microbiology (2008, June3), Humans Have Ten Times More Bacteria Than Human Cells. , *Science Daily*, http://www.sciencedaily.com/

21. Lewis Thomas *The Lives of a Cell: Notes of a Biology Watcher* (New York: Viking Press, 1974). Fascinating reading about the anomalies of living systems.

22. Brian Greene *The Fabric of the Cosmos: Space, Time, and the Texture of Reality* (New York: Random House, 2004). A good introduction to quantum mechanics, relativity, and cosmology.

23. Seth (2009, March 18), "Object and Process Oriented Languages and Human Development". *It's Elemental,* http://www.spiritalchemy.com/397/object-and-process-oriented-languages-and-human-development/

Chapter 6   Trading mental health for addiction

24. Alcoholics Anonymous *Pass It On: The Story of Bill Wilson and How the A.A. Message Reached the World* (New York: Alcoholics Anonymous World Services, 1984), p. 114. An incredible story well worth reading.

25. *Alcoholics Anonymous: The Big Book, 4th edition* (New York: Alcoholics Anonymous World Services, Inc., 2001).

26. James Lovelock *The Vanishing Face of Gaia* (New York: Basic Books, 2009).

Chapter 7   The commercialization of mental health

27. Marcia Angell *The Truth About Drug Companies: How They Deceive Us and What to Do About It* (New York: Random House, 2004).

28. Daniel Carlat *Unhinged: The Trouble with Psychiatry-A Doctor's Revelations* about *a Profession in Crisis* (New York: Free Press, 2010).

29. Ray Moynihan & Alan Cassels *Selling Sickness: How the World's Biggest Pharmaceutical Companies Are Turning Us All Into Patients* (New York: Nation Books, 2005).

30. John Abramson *Overdosed America* (New York: Harper Collins, 2004).

Chapter 8   The war on drugs

31. Joseph Perez (author), Janet Lloyd (translator) *The Spanish Inquisition: A History* (New Haven: Yale University Press, 2005).

32. Glen R. Hanson, Peter J. Venturelli, Annette E. Fleckenstein *Drugs and Society, Eleventh Edition* (Burlington, MA: Jones and Bartlett Learning. 2012). This book is an incredibly rich source of information about drug use and abuse from the biological, behavioral, and social perspectives.

33. Steven B. Duke and Albert C. Gross *America's Longest War: Rethinking Our Tragic Crusade Against Drugs* (New York: G. P. Putnam, 1994).

34. Dan Baum *Smoke and Mirrors: The War on Drugs and the Politics of Failure* (New York: Little, Brown and Company, 1996).

35. John H. Richardson "A Radical Solution To End the Drug War: Legalize Everything", in *Esquire,* September 1, 2009 (http://www.esquire.com/the-side/richardson-report/drug-war-facts-090109). The voice of experience-from a former cop.

36. William F. Buckley Jr. "The War on Drugs is Lost", in *National Review*, February 12, 1996 (http://old.nationalreview.com/12feb96/drug.html).

37. Drug Sense "Drug War Clock", in *DrugSense Map, Inc.,* February 29, 2012 (http://www.drugsense.org/cms/wodclock).

Chapter 9   Essential addiction and essential health

38. Mel B. *New Wine: The Spiritual Roots of the Twelve Step Miracle* (Center City, MN: Hazelden Publishing, 1991).

Chapter 10   Attention and peacefulness

39. Daniel Goleman *The Meditative Mind: The Varieties of Meditative Experience* (New York: Tarcher. 1988).

40. Lawrence LeShan *How to Meditate* (new York: Bantum, 1974).

41. Jon Kabat-Zinn *Wherever You Go, There You Are: Mindfulness Meditation in Everyday Life* (New York: Hyperion, 1994).

42. Walter V. Obajnyk *Gathering the Light: A Psychology of Meditation* (Boston: Shambala, 1993).

43. Shunryu Suzuki *Zen Mind, Beginner's Mind* (New York: **Weatherhill, 1970).**

Chapter 11   Changing Thinking, Habits, and Beliefs

44. Dean Radin *Entangled Minds: Extrasensory Experiences in a Quantum Reality* (New York: Pocket Books, 2006). Ties weird quantum physics together with parapsychology to provide new insights.

45. Sigmund Freud *Beyond the Pleasure Principle (The Standard Edition)* Trans., James Strachey (New York: Liveright Publishing Corp., 1961).

46. UNESCO "The Seville Statement on Violence, Spain 1986" (en.wikipedia.org/wiki/Seville_statement_on_violence).

47. Iain McGilchrist *The Master and his Emissary: The Divided Brain and the Making of the Western World* (New Haven: Yale University Press, 2009). Covers a massive amount of material gathered over many years.

Chapter 12   New life experience

48. Carl Jung *Man and his Symbols* (New York: Dell Publishing, 1964).

49. Clare Dunne *Carl Jung: Wounded Healer of the Soul: An Illustrated Biography* (London: Continuum International Publishing Group, 2002).
Not enough can be said about the genius of Carl Jung. He was exceptionally far ahead of his time in what he understood. He was not only a physician and a psychologist, but an anthropologist and philosopher of the first degree. He spent time with physicists just as the age of quantum physics was dawning; and he apparently foresaw the mergence of old and new which is happing today. Jung wrote so much that it is a major undertaking to read all of his original works. The study of his biographies is perhaps the most economical route to understanding his huge contribution to the world.

Daniel J. Thompson, Ph.D. is a clinical psychologist practicing in San Antonio, Texas for thirty-eight years. His primary areas of interest are addiction and holism. He has served on the faculties of Trinity University and Saint Mary's University, and has lectured and taught extensively in the San Antonio area. Daniel is in private practice as a psychotherapist and consultant serving individuals, couples, and families. He also is a certified specialist in the treatment of alcohol and substance use disorders.

8600 Wurzbach Road, Suite 1103
San Antonio, TX 78240

Phone (210) 822-5971

.

www.ingramcontent.com/pod-product-compliance
Lightning Source LLC
Chambersburg PA
CBHW050530280326
41933CB00011B/1527